MCQs in Pharmacy Practice

MCQs in Pharmacy Practice

Second edition

Edited by

Lilian M Azzopardi

BPharm (Hons), MPhil, PhD, MRPharmS

Associate Professor and Head of Department
Department of Pharmacy
University of Malta
Msida, Malta

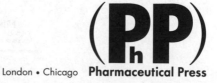

London • Chicago **Pharmaceutical Press**

Published by the Pharmaceutical Press

An imprint of RPS Publishing

1 Lambeth High Street, London SE1 7JN, UK
100 South Atkinson Road, Suite 200, Grayslake, IL 60030–7820, USA

© Pharmaceutical Press 2004, 2009

(P$_h$P) is a trade mark of RPS Publishing

RPS Publications is the publishing organisation of the Royal
Pharmaceutical Society of Great Britain

First published 2004
Second edition 2009

Typeset by J&L Composition, Scarborough, North Yorkshire
Printed in Great Britain by TJ International, Padstow, Cornwall

ISBN 978 0 85369 839 5

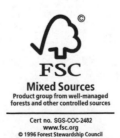

FSC

Mixed Sources
Product group from well-managed
forests and other controlled sources

Cert no. SGS-COC-2482
www.fsc.org
© 1996 Forest Stewardship Council

Contents

Foreword to the second edition

The International Pharmaceutical Federation (FIP) has stated: 'Maintaining competence throughout a career during which new and challenging professional responsibilities will be encountered is a fundamental ethical requirement for all health professionals. Patients have a right to be confident that professionals providing health care remain competent throughout their working lives.' (*Statement of Professional Standards on Continuing Professional Development*. The Hague: FIP, 2002.)

To become competent and effective pharmacists, there is a need for preregistration trainees and practising pharmacists to have a strong background knowledge as well as the ability to retrieve, to evaluate critically and to apply that knowledge in decision making. It is also important that, as part of the continuing professional development (CPD) process, pharmacists keep informed and continuously revise and assess their knowledge. Furthermore, during their career many pharmacists move from one sector of the profession to another or change their role within a particular sector. Pharmacists will need to update their knowledge in order to become competent and skilled practitioners in new areas.

Multiple choice questions are increasingly used to test knowledge and understanding objectively at an undergraduate level and in licensing exams. They can be formative as self-assessment exercises with feedback and are particularly useful for revision purposes and as a means of identifying an area for further study.

This book provides the reader with a variety of practice MCQs, which can be used to assess essential pharmacy practice knowledge in a number of areas, including drug action, uses, clinical pharmacology, adverse effects, pharmaceutical care, counselling points, product selection and pharmaceutical calculations. It will be a very useful text both for pharmacy preregistration examination candidates and for practising pharmacists.

Professor Claire Anderson
School of Pharmacy, Faculty of Science, University of Nottingham, United Kingdom
April 2009

Foreword to the first edition

To practise pharmacy effectively and accountably, it is critical for practitioners to have a sound, contemporary and comprehensive database. In addition to the many good references in textbooks and the periodical literature, there is a certain amount of knowledge that we have to keep current in our memory and daily dialogue. An appropriate balance must be struck by our reliance on memory and our capacity to find, analyse and apply useful knowledge to effective clinical decision making. Much discussion is currently ongoing around the world of the ideas captured in the phrase 'continuing professional development' (CPD). Simply put, CPD reflects the fact that, for pharmacy professionals to practise with responsibility and accountability, each one must structure a plan and implement mechanisms by which they can maintain their individual competence. It also indicates a willingness of the individual practitioner to build a portfolio of formal and informal educational processes in which they are continuously engaged to ensure competence. They are also willing to have this portfolio reviewed by their peers and perhaps, regulatory bodies, to establish a formal recognition of competence by external parties. Our profession will be examining these precepts over the coming years as a necessary evolution of our thinking around continuing education, public accountability and personal professional development.

Engaging in review of important developments in the field of pharmacy and the disciplines that support its knowledge system is a personal responsibility that all practitioners must take seriously.

This is particularly true at this time in the evolution of our profession. As we globally embrace the precepts of pharmaceutical care, as we find an appropriate balance between knowing our products, our patients and their disease states, it is increasingly critical to constantly review new findings as well as legacy principles. One way of doing that is self-assessment.

Shaping a personal way of assessing one's knowledge is an important commitment to continuous professional development and demonstration of personal competence. Self-assessment that is taken seriously has the capacity to identify areas where further 'sharpening' is needed. It also provides the capacity to validate what one knows related to the competence requirements of one's practice. Such assessment is not a comparison of what one knows compared with others but rather, focuses on the skills, knowledge and attitudes that are relevant to an individual's practice.

MCQs in Pharmacy Practice is an important effort to engage individual pharmacists in such self-assessment. The authors of this text have identified a way by which individual pharmacists, who are committed to their own continuing professional development, can apply a systematic way of involving themselves in self assessment.

This text provides a guided way of asking important questions, pointing out salient features of rational drug therapy and stimulating deeper thinking through a variety of exercises.

Pharmacists who work their way through this book will assuredly gain in their knowledge and skills. More importantly, they will be able to identify those areas in which they may need deeper study. But going through only this text will not ensure practice competence. The need to stay current with the contemporary literature, involving oneself in formal lecture programmes, being part of intra- and inter-professional scientific dialogue and myriad other ways in which one sharpens one's skills, will still be important engagements. By blending these

efforts with structured self-assessment, such as that offered by
MCQs in Pharmacy Practice, the individual practitioner will
have taken major steps in ensuring individual competence.

Henri R Manasse, Jr, BS, MA, PhD, ScD, RPh
Executive Vice President and Chief Executive Officer
American Society of Health-System Pharmacists,
Bethesda, Maryland, USA
December 2002

Preface to the second edition

The first edition of the book *MCQs in Pharmacy Practice* was published in 2004. This timeframe gave assessors of professionals practising in the health field time to follow the evolvement of the different forms of MCQs. Six years ago, adopting a multiple choice format as opposed to the traditional essay-type was a daring task with all its implications on how much fairer the new system was over the traditional one.

In this second edition, Lilian Azzopardi has succeeded to move further away from the True/False type of setting to more challenging formats. The newer types of MCQs demand appreciation of the subject whereby knowledge accrued is tested by having to judge whether the first of two statements is true and decision-making skills are required to decide whether the second statement is a correct explanation of the first. Another format which has the advantage not only of testing factual knowledge but also that of mimicking realistic clinical situations is where the student has not only to select the route or product to use but also to be able to indicate the next best option while identifying which other option would be least suitable. Such questions are ably set while still allowing for an unbiased assessment. The extension of the types of setting, albeit more demanding on the contributors, make the second edition of *MCQs in Pharmacy Practice* truly comprehensive in style. Such questions also provide the student with a refreshing exercise in mind juggling with pharmaceutical principles.

The BNF recommended for use with the first edition of *MCQs in Pharmacy Practice* was the 44th edition. At the time of writing this preface, the latest edition of the British National Formulary (BNF 57) was published. The editor has therefore updated the information in the questions to reflect that in the current BNF, so as to ensure that the questions are practical and contemporary. The answers given to the questions, which again form an essential part of this edition have been meticulously updated by Lilian M Azzopardi, recently appointed Head of Department of Pharmacy in the Faculty of Medicine and Surgery. In this capacity Lilian Azzopardi acts as chairperson of the examination boards in pharmacy practice including the final examination (which is in an MCQ format) that leads to registration as a pharmacist. As Dean of the Faculty of Medicine and Surgery, to which the department of pharmacy belongs, I could read in this text the meticulousness and diligence that are so characteristic of the attributes that Professor Azzopardi possesses.

Professor Godfrey LaFerla
Dean and Head of Department of Surgery, Faculty of
Medicine and Surgery, University of Malta
Chairman, Department of Surgery, Mater Dei Hospital, Malta
April 2009

Preface to the first edition

For many years pharmacy education was based on the study of a number of 'classic' basic and applied sciences such as chemistry, mathematics, pharmaceutics, pharmacognosy and pharmacology. Students were then examined separately in these different disciplines. It is only fairly recently that pharmacy practice and pharmaceutical care have been introduced as integral parts of the pharmacy curriculum. Attempts at finding the best way to test the competence of pharmacy students were made at roughly the same time.

Educationalists in many different disciplines have sought ways of testing objectively a student's knowledge of a subject. A perfectly fair examination is one in which students are objectively and accurately assessed with regard to their comprehension, analysis, evaluation and application of all the material with which they have been presented during their course of studies. Multiple choice questions have been accepted as such an objective measure in most areas, including those related to professional practice.

Pharmacy practice has, until very recently, been examined through the traditional essay type of question. This has led, at times, to the feeling that the overall assessment of this discipline could be a subjective one. The MCQ system tries to eliminate the subjective element in an examination and is now well established as a fair mode of assessment. The availability of a pharmacy practice text based on the MCQ system now provides pharmacy students with the opportunity of assessing themselves in the discipline and finding out whether they have mastered it. Dr Azzopardi and her collaborators are to be congratulated in having managed to produce this text. Dr Azzopardi's book has both breadth and depth and should test a student's knowledge rigorously. It should be a welcome addition to the standard texts students use during the years spent in training to become pharmacists.

Roger Ellul-Micallef
Rector, Professor and Head of Department
Clinical Pharmacology and Therapeutics,
University of Malta, Malta
December 2002

Introduction

The statement by John Biggs (*Teaching for Quality Learning at University*. Milton Keynes: Open University Press, 1999) that 'assessment drives student learning' is still as true today as it was in 1999 and can be applied equally to undergraduate learning and continuing professional development (CPD). In both areas, access to assessment tasks that allow for self-assessment of knowledge across a broad range of domains is important. *MCQs in Pharmacy Practice 2nd edn* contains a broad range of multiple-choice questions that provide feedback on what is known and where knowledge is lacking. This information is useful to many potential users — the pharmacy undergraduate, the preregistrant, the university professor and the practising pharmacist.

At all levels, understanding the limitations in our knowledge and abilities is a critical step in the learning process. Learning that is based on individual knowledge gaps is more likely to be effective and the learner is more motivated. The ability to identify one's own learning needs is often a challenging and time-consuming process, even though the results can be rewarding. *MCQs in Pharmacy Practice 2nd edn* is a simple-to-use, useful, unintimidating text that enables users to determine the extent of their knowledge, to identify knowledge gaps and to test their ability to analyse information and to make decisions.

This text is primarily aimed at preparing students to sit for multiple choice question (MCQ) examinations in pharmacy and would therefore be a valuable study tool for students preparing for registration and would also assist in preparation for other types of examination, such as oral examinations. It provides students and pharmacists with an excellent resource to test their knowledge and to highlight areas where they require further work.

In the undergraduate setting there are many opportunities throughout the curriculum for students and professors to utilise MCQs to assess knowledge in particular areas. *MCQs in Pharmacy Practice 2nd edn* would therefore make a useful prescribed text to guide self-directed study for undergraduate pharmacy students. Continual, regular assessment of students provides a form of feedback to students on the level of knowledge gained and areas where additional work is needed. This text would be of equal value if sections of the text were given to students as regular formative assessment or if students used the text as a study guide.

The primary aim of professional development in pharmacy is to develop and maintain competencies, which improve standards of care and health outcomes for patients. Knowledge is a critical element in this process and community pharmacists invest significant time and money undertaking CPD. One of the major barriers to effective CPD is motivation to undertake further learning reflected in reasons given for lack of engagement with CPD, such as lack of time, cost and lack of engagement with educational formats. A contributing factor to this lack of engagement is the inability to match individual learning needs with educational offerings. These questions provide an excellent tool to enable practising pharmacists to assess their own knowledge in a variety of relevant areas. Once gaps in knowledge are identified, it is a simpler process to undertake self-directed learning that addresses deficiencies and CPD is therefore more stimulating and meaningful and likely to lead to a change in practice.

Multiple choice questions are time consuming and difficult to develop in a manner that ensures appropriate assessment of knowledge and critical thinking skills. The questions in *MCQs in Pharmacy Practice 2nd edn* are of an excellent standard and the format, variety and structure make it an essential resource for the pharmacy profession.

Associate Professor Jennifer Marriott
Director, Bachelor of Pharmacy Course, Faculty of
Pharmacy and Pharmaceutical Sciences, Monash University,
Australia
President, Academic Section, International
Pharmaceutical Federation

Acknowledgements

I would like to thank colleagues and friends who have supported me in completing the second edition of this book. I am most grateful to the contributing authors: Anthony Serracino-Inglott and Maurice Zarb Adami from the University of Malta, Steve Hudson from the University of Strathclyde and Sam Salek from the University of Cardiff. I would like to thank pharmacists Alison Anastasi and Louise Azzopardi for their participation in reviewing the material. Gratitude is also due to Juanito Camilleri, Rector, and Godfrey Laferla, Dean of the Faculty of Medicine and Surgery, University of Malta for their constant support.

Thanks also go to staff and students at the Department of Pharmacy especially Amanda Calleja and staff at the Faculty of Medicine and Surgery. I would like to acknowledge the assistance received from staff at Pharmaceutical Press, particularly Christina DeBono and Louise McIndoe.

About the editor

Lilian M Azzopardi studied pharmacy at the University of Malta, Faculty of Medicine and Surgery. In 1994 she took up a position at the Department of Pharmacy, University of Malta as a teaching and research assistant. Professor Azzopardi completed an MPhil on the development of formulary systems for community pharmacy in 1995, and in 1999 she gained a PhD. Her thesis led to the publication of the book *Validation Instruments for Community Pharmacy: pharmaceutical care for the third millennium* published in 2000 by Pharmaceutical Products Press, USA. She worked together with Professor Anthony Serracino Inglott who was a pioneer in the introduction of clinical pharmacy in the late sixties. Professor Azzopardi is the author of *Further MCQs In Pharmacy Practice (2006)* and *MCQs in Clinical Pharmacy* (2007) by Pharmaceutical Press.

Professor Azzopardi is currently an associate professor in pharmacy practice at the Department of Pharmacy, University of Malta and is responsible for coordinating several aspects of teaching of pharmacy practice, including clinical pharmacy for undergraduate and postgraduate students, as well as supervising a number of pharmacy projects and dissertations in the field. She is an examiner at the University of Malta for students following the course of pharmacy and is an assessor in determining suitability to practice.

Lilian Azzopardi was for a short period interim director of the European Society of Clinical Pharmacy (ESCP) and is currently coordinator of the ESCP newsletter. She served as a member of the Working Group on Quality Care Standards within the Community Pharmacy Section of the International Pharmaceutical Federation (FIP). She was a member of the Pharmacy Board, the licensing authority for pharmacy in Malta for a number of years and Registrar of the Malta College of Pharmacy Practice, which is responsible for continuing education. In 1997 she received an award from the FIP Foundation for Education and Research and in 1999 gained the ESCP German Research and Education Foundation grant. She has practised clinical pharmacy in the hospital setting and she practises in community pharmacy.

Lilian Azzopardi has published several papers on clinical pharmacy and pharmaceutical care and has actively participated at congresses organised by FIP, ESCP, RPSGB, APhA and ASHP. She has been invited to give lectures and short courses in this area in several universities. She has been a member of scientific committees for European conferences and chaired a number of oral communication sessions reporting research work in the field of pharmacy practice. She has received funding for her research projects from national institutions and in 2008 completed a project funded by the European Union on automated dispensing of pharmaceuticals and pharmacist interventions, of which she was project coordinator for the University of Malta. In 2008 Professor Azzopardi was appointed head of the department of pharmacy at the University of Malta.

Contributors

Lilian M Azzopardi BPharm (Hons), MPhil, PhD, MRPharmS
Associate Professor and Head of Department, Department of Pharmacy, Faculty of Medicine and Surgery, University of Malta, Msida, Malta

Stephen A Hudson MPharm, FRPharmS
Professor of Pharmaceutical Care, Division of Pharmaceutical Sciences, University of Strathclyde Institute of Pharmacy and Biomedical Sciences, University of Strathclyde, UK

Sam Salek PhD, RPh, MFPM (Hon)
Professor and Director, Centre for Socioeconomic Research, Welsh School of Pharmacy, Cardiff University, UK

Anthony Serracino-Inglott BPharm, PharmD, MRPharmS
Professor, Department of Pharmacy, University of Malta, Msida, Malta

Maurice Zarb-Adami BPharm, BPharm(Lond), PhD
Senior Lecturer, Department of Pharmacy, University of Malta, Msida, Malta

How to use this book

This book provides an ideal revision guide for those preparing to sit for a multiple choice questions (MCQs) examination in pharmacy. It covers common general pharmacy practice interventions and operations and other topics commonly featured in examinations, such as simple pharmaceutical calculations, doses, strengths, nomenclature, abbreviations, dosage forms, specialities, trade and generic names, biochemical tests, classification, side-effects, and common diseases. Some recent advances in pharmacy practice are also included.

It is recommended that students use this book in their final preparatory stage before sitting for qualifying, licensing or registration examinations so that they are aware of the nature of the questions likely to be posed and how best to approach the examination. This series of MCQ tests is aimed at preparing candidates for their registration examination, whether this is carried out by the state board, the pharmaceutical society or the university. In setting out a broad range of typical MCQs, the aim is to test the level of the candidate's knowledge, as well as helping to reinforce specific points and refine the examination technique.

This book consists of 800 examination-type MCQs (300 of which are new questions and over 30 new drug entities are included). The questions are practice oriented and are intended to assess knowledge, evaluative and analytical skills, and ability to apply that knowledge in clinical practice.

The book consists of two parts. The first is an open-book section wherein the questions aim to assess the student's ability to apply their knowledge in a practice setting in conjunction with the use of information sources. In the second part, the closed-book section, MCQs are directed towards basic skills and knowledge with which the student is expected to be fully familiar.

Each test consists of 100 questions which should be completed in two hours. In each test, different formats of MCQs are adopted. Each format is introduced with directions for answering the MCQs. In each test, case-based and free-standing questions are included. Answers with brief explanations are given at the end of each test.

For each test, write the number of the question and your answer on a separate sheet of paper, then after going through all the questions in the test, compare your answers with those in the book. Attempt one open-book test and one closed-book test so as to mimic examination conditions. Refer to Appendix D for feedback on those questions you did not answer correctly. Information on the proprietary names listed in the book is given in Appendix A. Appendix B includes definitions of medical terms included in the book, while Appendix C lists abbreviations and acronyms.

The recommended textbooks for the open-book section are:

Azzopardi LM (2000). *Validation Instruments for Community Pharmacy: Pharmaceutical Care for the Third Millennium.* Binghamton, New York: Pharmaceutical Products Press.

Edwards C, Stillman P (2006). *Minor Illness or Major Disease? The Clinical Pharmacist in the Community*, 4th edn. London: Pharmaceutical Press.

Joint Formulary Committee (2009). *British National Formulary*, London: Pharmaceutical Press.

Medicines, Ethics and Practice: a Guide for Pharmacists and Pharmacy Technicians, 32, July 2008. London: Royal Pharmaceutical Society of Great Britain, 2008.

Nathan A (2006). *Non-prescription Medicines*, 3rd edn. London: Pharmaceutical Press.

This book is mainly meant for those sitting the final test before being registered as pharmacists. This test is considered to be one of the most challenging tasks in a student's training. The syllabus and specific requirements regarding eligibility to sit for the examination have been carefully laid down by the relevant authorities but the aim is always the same: namely, an attempt to set the required standards of professional skills and ability. The format of the examination itself has been selected to test these standards thoroughly. These preregistration examinations are a necessary obstacle to overcome in becoming a professional pharmacist, in whose hands patients are safe and who is a credit to the profession.

The MCQs method of assessing students is here to stay. MCQs are no longer regarded as an examination that constitutes a final handshake for those who have completed four years at university, passed all the tests, practised in the pharmacy service, gained experience and have received a good report from their mentor pharmacist. Indeed, a poor performance in this assessment may result in overall failure.

MCQs in pharmacy practice do not simply examine facts. Some students expect MCQs to test only factual knowledge. However, questions are also set to test the candidate's ability to comprehend the statements, analyse them and give a logical answer. Some MCQs also test the ability to make safe clinical decisions, and occasionally even test the candidate's professional bearing.

Thorough preparation for an MCQs examination is essential — the information gained and stored during pharmacy practice sessions carried out in a pharmaceutical environment will form the foundation of the candidates' knowledge to enable them to pass the examination.

Preparing and sitting for MCQs in pharmacy practice

Advice about answering MCQs is not very different from that for any other examination, whether oral or written. Starting with dress, there is a tendency to match your psychological outlook and actions to the way you are dressed. Some students approach MCQ tests casually, as if this type of examination were not as serious an undertaking as any other. Dress smartly but comfortably and conservatively. Avoid clothes that make you feel too relaxed, such as casual jackets or leisure wear.

Arrive a little early for the examination and plan how much time to allocate for each question, allowing extra time for more difficult questions.

Open-book examinations

The rarity of absolutes in pharmacy practice means that a variety of adjectives and adverbs are commonly used in its description, increasing the difficulty of answering MCQs. Although the desirability of assessing knowledge that is dependent on the 'strength' of an adjective can be questioned, these adjectives do form part of the language of present-day pharmacy practice, borne out by their frequent use in the questions and answers presented in this book. You should not assume they are clues — they may or may not be.

The following are suggestions about how to tackle the questions in Test 1 of this book. These pointers may be applied to the other tests in this publication. The questions are tackled in groups and a number of points are considered. However, some of the points discussed may certainly be adopted in answering other questions. Sometimes the open-book questions may even present more of a challenge than the closed-book questions. In the case of Test 1, which is an open-book examination, there is also advice about the best use of reference books within the time allowed for answering the MCQs.

Questions 1–25

Several questions contain the statement: 'All … EXCEPT'. In this book, 'except' is in capital letters (upper case) but not all texts use this convention. More important is the fact that only *one* answer — *one* choice — is allowed. This is explained in the statement at the beginning of the questions.

Never underestimate the importance of reading the directions very carefully. In this case, the directions state: 'Select the best answer in each case.' (Note the use of the word 'best'.) Do not spend too much time, however, selecting the 'best' answer — very often there is only one *correct* answer. Candidates who select more than one answer will not be given any marks, even if the choice includes the correct answer.

Another type of question includes the word 'NOT' — again this book uses upper case but this may not be so in all examinations, so watch out for such words (for example, in Q4).

Do not be unduly perturbed by the word 'appropriate' when it is stated that there is only one correct answer. The chances are that there is only one 'therapeutic alternative' (Q6). 'Appropriate' is used only as a linguistic necessity because, if it were omitted, then the other alternatives might be possible, if not appropriate. In practice, however, no other 'alternative' is available except the correct answer. 'Appropriate' is therefore superfluous and should not bother you. Focus more on the term 'bedridden', which is an indication of possible long-term use of the laxative (Q8).

The same applies to 'optimum' in Q12. There is only one correct range for plasma theophylline concentrations. 'Optimum' here is again a nicety of the language.

Be careful about the use of 'over-the-counter', which actually means 'without a prescription'. Note that the emphasis is rarely on 'over-the-counter' but on the condition. In Q13 the term is again superfluous and you should not be confused by it. 'Over-the-counter' is often introduced to denote that this is a pharmacy practice examination and therefore the exceptional use of substances indicated only in very rare cases is excluded.

Similarly, 'because' means a description of an action of a drug and so, in questions such as Q14, the importance of the drug rather than the disease should be stressed. However, if you do not know the action of the specific drug then a good suggestion would be to look at the disease and examine what action is required to address the particular ailment.

Other terms are used, such as 'differs', which does not necessarily mean 'different from'; in Q20 the question refers to a *total* difference in the components of the products. 'Equivalent to' usually means having the same active ingredients, or a drug belonging to the same class, and not equivalent in 'use' or in 'action' (Q23).

MCQs, contrary to what some students fear, are not meant to be tricky. Do not try to read between the lines but do read the statements very carefully. Many mistakes happen because the directions are not carefully followed. This kind of exercise is part of the test itself, as in pharmacy practice, mistakes are often made because a prescription or the patient's drug profile have not been properly read.

Questions 26–52

The tests are set so that there are 100 questions with an open-book option, and another 100 questions of the closed-book type. Questions in both formats may appear to be complex in their setting. Devote enough time to understand the question clearly. Statements or advice that a heading may be used once, more than once or not at all mean exactly that.

The term 'most closely related to' (*see* directions for Q26–52) is not a 'trick' and you should not expect to find some statements more closely related than others. Very often only one statement is obviously related and it is safe to assume that the other answers are incorrect. Do not be misled by the use of 'most closely', which is actually superfluous.

In an open-book situation, expect a number of proprietary (trade) names or diseases. Although candidates are allowed to look up all the trade names in the textbooks available, in an examination this is not practical and sometimes impossible to achieve in the allocated time. Check the active ingredients of a proprietary name only when necessary or when in doubt. You are expected to have a good knowledge of most brands and pharmaceutical manufacturers (Q26–40).

Diseases tend to present a distinct challenge to pharmacy practice examination candidates. Students often do their best to gain as much knowledge of drugs as possible, but when it comes to diseases they are confused. There are so many thousands of diseases, where should one start? Which diseases should be revised for an MCQs examination? What depth of knowledge about diseases is expected? In tackling these questions it is important to be very familiar with the textbooks used in the open-book examination. Very often the rule of thumb is 'the simpler, the better', so do *not* take encyclopaedias with you to the examination. A book such as *Martindale: the Complete Drug Reference* may be useful but it is not essential and would only be used on a few occasions. However, a reference such as the *British National Formulary* (BNF) should be kept at hand. For this edition, the 57th edition (March 2009) was used.

Let us examine how, for example, Q32–34 could be tackled by the following steps:

1   Write the generic names next to A—E, starting with those that you are confident about.
2   Find the ones you do not know, or are unsure of, in the BNF index (at this stage, just note the page numbers).
3   Find the generic names by going through the pages, checking the list in alphabetical order, rather than going backwards and forwards, to save time.

(Any reference books to be used in the examination should not be bought at the last moment — books should have been used for some time because it is easier to turn the pages, as those in new books tend to stick together; such minor annoyances encountered during an examination can increase the tension. In addition, get used to the newer editions of the textbooks. Practise using the indexes, appendices and footnotes and be familiar with the overall structure of the reference books used in an open-book session.)

The phrase 'associated with' used, for example, in Q35–37, means only 'who is the manufacturer of that particular drug?' This information should not be sought, say, in a pharmacology textbook but can be easily located in a formulary such as the BNF.

First write the page numbers next to Q35–37, after finding them in the index (preferably in alphabetical order to save time) and then find the corresponding pages in the text. You will find the manufacturer's name in parentheses next to the product name.

Although in Q32–34 you only had to look for the products A—E and match them with the specific diseases, in Q35–37, do not attempt to find the manufacturers A—E; look up the three products instead. Q38–40 should be attempted in the same way as Q32–34.

Practise these simple techniques, although they seem obvious when you know about them, as this type of question can cause confusion when met unawares and could be a challenge even to the diligent student who studied the facts but who had no practice with MCQs.

The next group of questions refers more to diseases and biochemical tests (Q41–44). These questions present more of a problem, not because of their difficulty but owing to the technique needed to make the best use of the reference books available. In this case follow these steps:

1   Write the page numbers next to the choices A—E after consulting a drug index or formulary that you know

carries precautions to be taken with the use of drugs, e.g. the BNF.

2   Write in summary format the biochemical test/disease mentioned in these questions, namely: (Q41) liver function tests; (Q42) epilepsy; (Q43) thyroid function; (Q44) peptic ulcer.

3   In the BNF, look under cautions for levodopa — the second one listed is peptic ulceration, so put A next to Q44. For domperidone, there are only three lines of cautions, none listing any of the four conditions, so go straight on to consider fluvastatin. (When consulting the index, always note down and look up the page marked in bold first.) Under cautions for all statins, in the first few lines there is a statement advising a liver function test. In an examination, if you are pressed for time, do not continue reading all the cautions but move on immediately to the next drug after marking C next to Q41.

A good reminder is that a reference book in an open-book examination should be used just to support your knowledge and only in rare cases to find unknown data. The availability of books in an examination does not replace the need for studying, particularly basic facts that require instant recall. Lack of this kind of preparation is often one of the reasons why some candidates perform worse in an open-book examination than in a closed-book one. Do not expect to gather all the information during the examination — the questions are designed to ensure that only students who are well versed and properly trained in pharmacy practice will pass.

Questions 53–83

These questions (Q53–83), which present a choice of answers grouped together, are a common format that sometimes perplexes students. The system is not meant to confuse but is used to facilitate the marking procedure. In this book the directions are summarised in a box but this may not always be the case in examinations set by different boards. Follow these steps to answer this type of question:

1   Summarise the directions if not already presented this way.
2   Mark the correct statements as if they were true/false answers.
3   Collate the answers.
4   Match the collated answers with the letters A—E, as indicated in the directions.
5   Write your chosen letter next to the question.

Do not answer the questions by writing '1, 2' or '1, 2, 3' or 'T' or 'F' but follow the instructions exactly and put a letter A—E. The reverse is also true, that is, if you are asked to write numbers (in a rare case) or T and F, do not create your own summary.

Remember that answer papers are sometimes corrected by clerks, who are given strict rules for recording correct answers, which they are obliged to follow. More commonly today, the analysis is undertaken by computer, so not following the instructions may result in the answer being marked as incorrect, no matter what was written. In Test 1 in this book, for example, Q53–83, i.e. 30% of the examination, are given in this format. There have been reports that some students lost 30% of their marks simply because they did not follow the instructions.

It must be emphasised that, although all the information required to answer the questions correctly is available in the recommended textbooks, do not try to verify all the information.

In Q58, for example, you need to read the question carefully — in this case, the emphasis is on the word 'daily'. The information can be found in the BNF under 'monitoring' but it is time consuming to read it all very carefully and, in this type of question, it is better to spend more time carefully examining the statements, rather than browsing through the books. This is totally different from using the book to check a dosage regimen, a proprietary name or a caution.

Similarly in Q55 the word 'care' should not be confused with a contraindication. The BNF states under cautions: 'Reduce dose in the elderly'. This should be interpreted that care should be taken with the use of digoxin. You may ask — should care not be taken with the use of *all* medicines, especially in the elderly? In this context, the word 'care' should be taken as meaning with *special* care or caution.

Questions 58–63 refer to diseases. In addition to using formularies such as the BNF, in this case, you may need to refer to other textbooks such as *Minor Illness or Major Disease* (*see* Bibliography) to answer these types of questions. In tackling Q61, the emphasis that the textbook places on detection combing for head lice signifies that this is the diagnostic process. This indicates how important it is that an authoritative book is used in an examination when you are allowed a choice of textbooks. The use of such books will help you find the correct answer, even when the answer is not specifically stated as such but needs to be inferred. The textbook selected for use in open-book MCQs should have an extensive index for quick reference.

In Q63, dealing with tinea pedis, a glance at the index of a good textbook will immediately remind you that this is athlete's foot. Many textbooks give a summary but sometimes it is worth going beyond this. The whole text on the topic itself is, in some cases, only a short paragraph. In dealing with Q63, for example, if you restrict yourself to the summary, you may miss the fact that the maceration is white, as the description of the earlier stage of tinea pedis is described in the summary as a 'red eruption' in *Minor Illness or Major Disease*.

Questions 64–71 concern drug use, contraindications, cautions and side-effects, which may all be found in formularies such as the BNF. It is important to look under the drug names rather than try to find information by looking for a disease or symptom.

Some questions may take the form of a case study (Q72). These should be analysed as if the patient were presenting at the pharmacy. In this case, start with the diagnosis — here it is clearly a case of verruca. Once this step has been taken, the correct diagnosis can be confirmed by quick reference to a note on verrucas given, for example, in *Minor Illness or Major Disease*.

Questions 84–88

Questions 84–88 appear to be more complex than the rest. The choices C, D or E are simple true or false answers to the statements. The choice between A and B, however, depends on whether the second statement is an explanation of the first statement. In this book, the questions in this section carry clear directions and even a summary to help you understand how to tackle them. This may not be the case in all board examinations, so practise how to summarise complex directions.

The aim of the questions is to test your ability to reach logical conclusions. The correctness of the statements can be verified in the textbooks but the logic of the sequence cannot. This type of question is becoming more popular with examiners because it tests an important aspect of pharmacy practice, namely logical argument from data that can be extracted from books but which then has to be interpreted in the practical setting.

Questions 89–100

The dispensing of prescriptions is considered to be a primary function in pharmacy practice. This is tackled in the final part of the test (Q89–94). The statements on Xenical can all be found in the BNF, except for the one stating that it 'may be administered twice daily'. The answer to this part is in the prescription presented (bd) in the question itself. This instance is a clear example pointing to the need to read the prescription carefully (Q89–90).

In the case of the prescription relating to Daktacort (Q91–94), for candidates not familiar with its use, it is important to identify the active ingredients. Daktacort is listed in the BNF under hydrocortisone but its main use is as an antifungal agent.

The need to apply the cream sparingly results from the steroid content and its use twice rather than three times daily comes from the information on the prescription (bd).

Some proprietary names may not be familiar to certain candidates, because an effort has been made to make this book suitable for different countries. If you do not recognise the brand name, use Appendix A, where the active ingredients of all proprietary products listed in the book are included. Day Nurse, for example (Q6), is not listed in the BNF but you can find information about it in Appendix A.

Finally, to conclude these pointers on the open-book questions, let us look at the statistics for Test 1 presented in Appendix D. These statistics were recorded following the tests carried out by a sample of final-year students after a five-year university course which included the preregistration period. In Test 1, the questions that were answered incorrectly by the highest number of students were 54, 58, 61, 62 and 86, whereas the ones most often answered correctly were 1, 14, 17, 22, 25, 26, 27, 29, 30, 32, 33, 39, 45, 60, 67, 68, 81, 89, 91 and 98. Questions answered incorrectly were often those that required some logical thinking. A good lesson to conclude this section, therefore, is that no textbook should replace logical thinking, even during an open-book examination.

Closed-book examinations

Most of the advice given for the open-book examinations should also be kept in mind for the closed-book tests. It is essential to revise the major classes of drugs, comparing the use, unwanted effects, contraindications and alternative products available. In this section, Test 5 is used as the example to highlight the following areas for quick revision:

- cautionary labels (Q2)
- adverse effects (Q4, Q27)
- calculations (Q6, Q11, Q13, Q17, Q18, Q20, Q28)
- contraindications (Q7)
- drug interactions (Q8)
- pregnancy (Q9, Q80)
- extemporaneous preparations (Q3)
- disease management and drug indications (Q1, Q14, Q38; *see* Appendix B for short descriptions of diseases)
- drug classification (Q12, Q16, Q56)
- aetiology of disease (Q19)
- drug indications (Q25, Q26, Q29)
- drug actions (Q24, Q45–48)
- drug formulation (Q34, Q49)
- abbreviations (Q42–44; *see* Appendix C)
- disease symptoms (Q39–41, Q53; *see* Appendix B)
- predisposing factors and risk factors (Q54, Q65)
- prophylaxis (Q57)
- pharmacist interventions (Q75).

A good look at the index of this book indicates the items commonly encountered in examinations. The index is an exhaustive one and is divided into proprietary names, generic names, subject areas and conditions. A self-assessment exercise is to check that you have adequate knowledge of examples of the topics listed above and then attempt the tests. A review of the drugs in the index provides examples of medicines that certainly need attention. You should be familiar with the action, classification, side-effects, clinically significant drug interactions, contraindications and cautions of a number of classes of drugs, such as:

- antibacterials (e.g. penicillins, cephalosporins, cipro-floxacin, metronidazole, doxycycline)
- analgesics (e.g. codeine, tramadol, co-proxamol, paraceta-mol, non-steroidal anti-inflammatory drugs)
- vitamins and minerals (e.g. iron, folic acid, vitamin A, C, E, B12)
- cardiovascular drugs (e.g. thiazide diuretics, digoxin, beta-adrenoceptor blocking drugs, calcium-channel blockers, drugs acting on the renin—angiotensin system)
- antidiabetic (e.g. glibenclamide, gliclazide, metformin, insulin)
- gastrointestinal drugs (e.g. antacids, proton pump inhibitors, laxatives)
- anti-asthmatic therapy (e.g. bronchodilators, corticos-teroids)

Using the index it is possible to gain an insight into the selection of drugs covered in such examinations. Check that you know the meaning of the conditions listed in Appendix B and make lists of medicines that are indicated and contraindicated or that may precipitate the condition.

Finally, examining the statistics for Test 4 regarding questions that were answered incorrectly by the largest number of candidates, it can be concluded that nothing can replace practical observation during the in-service training in a pharmacy, for example, knowledge of the expiration date of extemporaneous preparations is information that is acquired during practice sessions (Q3). The use of medicines for prophylaxis, rather than for treatment, is often confused by candidates, as can be seen from the statistics for Q59, where allopurinol was mistaken for *treatment* of gout when it is indicated for *prophylactic* use. Some questions require reasoning rather than just recall of information, such as Q80 and Q90–92, Q93. Practise reasoning out answers when undertaking self-assessment questions before the examination.

Questions 5, 8, 12, 17, 22, 26, 39, 42, 43, 44, 46, 49, 61, 70, 72, 79, 85, 86, 88 and 95 were answered incorrectly by less than 5% of the candidates. It is advisable to tackle these questions first, as they ought to be answered easily, allowing more time for the questions where reasoning is required. Appendix D indicates which questions were the hardest. This should serve as a guide and can give feedback on how you would compare with colleagues in a qualifying or licensing and registration examination.

Note

Use of names for medicinal substances

The recommended International Non-proprietary Name (rINN) is used throughout the book, except when the terms used are adrenaline and noradrenaline. For further reference, see the *British National Formulary*.

Dosage forms

In the answers to questions and in Appendix A, when no mention of a dosage form (e.g. tablets, lotion, drops) is made, the data refer to the dosage form indicated in the questions.

Section 1

Open-book Questions

Test 1

Questions

Questions 1–25

Directions: Each of the questions or incomplete statements is followed by five suggested answers. Select the best answer in each case.

Q1 All of the following products contain hydrocortisone EXCEPT:

A ❑ Fucidin H
B ❑ Daktacort
C ❑ Fucicort
D ❑ Otosporin
E ❑ Canesten HC

Q2 All of the following accompanying symptoms for headache warrant referral EXCEPT:

A ❑ loss of consciousness
B ❑ neck stiffness
C ❑ paraesthesia
D ❑ slurred speech
E ❑ fever

Q3 Nifedipine:

A ❑ constricts vascular smooth muscle
B ❑ long-acting formulations are preferred in the long-term treatment of hypertension
C ❑ is a nitrate
D ❑ interferes with the inward displacement of potassium ions through active cell membranes
E ❑ results in increased risk of bradycardia when administered concomitantly with atenolol

Q4   Which of the following is NOT involved in the presentation of seasonal allergic rhinitis?

   A ❑ leukotrienes
   B ❑ prostaglandins
   C ❑ osteocytes
   D ❑ basophils
   E ❑ mast cells

Q5   Patient medication records should include all EXCEPT:

   A ❑ medication allergies
   B ❑ diagnosis
   C ❑ current medication therapy
   D ❑ pets kept at home
   E ❑ age

Q6   What is an appropriate therapeutic alternative for Uniflu?

   A ❑ Actifed
   B ❑ Day Nurse
   C ❑ Phenergan
   D ❑ Ventolin
   E ❑ Xyzal

Q7   Symptoms of vaginal candidiasis that warrant referral include all EXCEPT:

   A ❑ vaginal discharge
   B ❑ abdominal pain
   C ❑ fever
   D ❑ diabetes
   E ❑ pregnancy

Q8   An appropriate laxative preparation for an elderly patient who is bedridden is:

A   ❑ bisacodyl
B   ❑ senna
C   ❑ magnesium sulphate
D   ❑ lactulose
E   ❑ liquid paraffin

Q9   All of the following drugs affect the renin—angiotensin system EXCEPT:

A   ❑ hydralazine
B   ❑ valsartan
C   ❑ losartan
D   ❑ perindopril
E   ❑ lisinopril

Q10   A significant clinical interaction may occur if lithium is administered concomitantly with:

A   ❑ paroxetine
B   ❑ glibenclamide
C   ❑ co-amoxiclav
D   ❑ atenolol
E   ❑ nifedipine

Q11   Celecoxib:

A   ❑ is as effective as diclofenac
B   ❑ provides protection against ischaemic cardiovascular events
C   ❑ is indicated for long-term use in osteoarthritis
D   ❑ is not contraindicated in patients with cerebrovascular disease
E   ❑ is marketed under the proprietary name Mobic

Q12 For optimum response, plasma theophylline concentration should be maintained at:

A ❑ 30–40 mg/L
B ❑ 2–5 mg/L
C ❑ 8–10 mg/L
D ❑ 10–20 mg/L
E ❑ 20–25 mg/L

Q13 Appropriate preparations that could be dispensed over-the-counter to treat motion sickness include all of the following EXCEPT:

A ❑ Stugeron
B ❑ Avomine
C ❑ Kwells
D ❑ Motilium
E ❑ Phenergan

Q14 Alfuzosin is used in benign prostatic hyperplasia because it:

A ❑ lowers blood pressure
B ❑ decreases urinary flow rate
C ❑ constricts smooth muscle
D ❑ increases bladder capacity
E ❑ relaxes smooth muscle

Q15 Which of the following antibacterial agents is not presented for systemic use?

A ❑ sodium fusidate
B ❑ vancomycin
C ❑ gentamicin
D ❑ mupirocin
E ❑ doxycycline

Q16 All of the following products are Controlled Drugs EXCEPT:

A ❏ pethidine
B ❏ diazepam
C ❏ morphine
D ❏ alfentanil
E ❏ remifentanil

Q17 Famciclovir is:

A ❏ an ester of aciclovir
B ❏ too toxic for systemic use
C ❏ a pro-drug of penciclovir
D ❏ not indicated in acute genital herpes simplex
E ❏ indicated for the prophylaxis of varicella zoster

Q18 All of the following factors could precipitate the onset of herpes labialis EXCEPT:

A ❏ common cold
B ❏ sun
C ❏ trauma to the lips
D ❏ dental caries
E ❏ immunosuppression

Q19 The human papilloma virus vaccine Gardasil:

A ❏ may be administered to females from 9 years onwards
B ❏ eliminates the need for routine cervical screening
C ❏ is administered by intramuscular injection as a single dose
D ❏ is a bivalent vaccine
E ❏ requires the administration of 5 doses for a complete course

Q20   Cilest differs from Yasmin in that it:

   A   ❑   is used in hormone replacement therapy
   B   ❑   is available for transdermal drug delivery
   C   ❑   has to be taken twice daily
   D   ❑   contains norgestimate
   E   ❑   can be used in patients with venous thromboembolic disease

Q21   What is the most appropriate treatment that could be dispensed over-the-counter for irritation caused by contact dermatitis?

   A   ❑   Eurax cream
   B   ❑   Canesten HC cream
   C   ❑   Hydrocortisone cream
   D   ❑   Clarityn tablets
   E   ❑   Pevaryl cream

Q22   Which of the following products is NOT indicated for the treatment of insomnia?

   A   ❑   Stilnoct
   B   ❑   diazepam
   C   ❑   Heminevrin
   D   ❑   Buspar
   E   ❑   Phenergan

Q23   Which of the following products may be recommended as an equivalent to Rhinocort Aqua?

   A   ❑   Molcer
   B   ❑   Otrivine
   C   ❑   Nasonex
   D   ❑   Emadine
   E   ❑   Sudafed

Q24   Bupivacaine:

A   ❏ has a rapid onset of action
B   ❏ is suitable for continuous epidural analgesia in labour
C   ❏ is of short duration of action
D   ❏ is used in dentistry
E   ❏ is presented in Xylocaine

Q25   Haloperidol is used in the treatment of all of the following conditions EXCEPT:

A   ❏ motor tics
B   ❏ schizophrenia
C   ❏ intractable hiccup
D   ❏ parkinsonism
E   ❏ severe anxiety

Questions 26–52

Directions: Each group of questions below consists of five lettered headings followed by a list of numbered questions. For each numbered question select the one heading that is most closely related to it. Each heading may be used once, more than once, or not at all.

Questions 26–28 concern the following vaccines:

A   ❏ Twinrix
B   ❏ Rotarix
C   ❏ Engerix B
D   ❏ Fluarix
E   ❏ Havrix

Select, from A to E, which one of the above:

Q26   covers against hepatitis A and B

Q27   is a live attenuated vaccine available for oral administration

Q28   contains the H and N component of the prevalent strains as indicated by the World Health Organization

Questions 29–31 concern the following products:

A   ❑ Zinnat
B   ❑ Zofran
C   ❑ Cytotec
D   ❑ Indocid
E   ❑ Diamox

Select, from A to E, the product that can cause:

Q29   constipation

Q30   abnormal vaginal bleeding

Q31   paraesthesia

Questions 32–34 concern the following products:

A   ❑ Cardura
B   ❑ Inderal
C   ❑ Cozaar
D   ❑ Tildiem
E   ❑ Aldactone

Select, from A to E, the product that should be used with caution in the following conditions:

Q32   porphyria

Q33   diabetes

Q34   myasthenia gravis

Questions 35–37 concern the following manufacturers:

A   ❑   AstraZeneca
B   ❑   Schering-Plough
C   ❑   Boehringer Ingelheim
D   ❑   Lilly
E   ❑   Abbott

Select, from A to E, which one of the above manufacturers is associated with the trademarked product:

Q35   Byetta

Q36   Nexium

Q37   Alupent

Questions 38–40 concern the following products:

A   ❑   Karvol
B   ❑   Rynacrom
C   ❑   Difflam
D   ❑   Molcer
E   ❑   Daktarin

Select, from A to E, the product that is presented in the following dosage forms:

Q38   oral rinse

Q39   nasal spray

Q40   ear drops

Questions 41–44 concern the following drugs:

A ❏ levodopa
B ❏ domperidone
C ❏ fluvastatin
D ❏ lithium
E ❏ fluvoxamine

Select, from A to E, which of the above:

Q41   should prompt liver function tests before initiating treatment

Q42   should be used with caution in patients with epilepsy

Q43   requires monitoring of thyroid function

Q44   should be used with caution in patients with diabetes mellitus

Questions 45–48 concern the following strengths:

A ❏ 2 mg
B ❏ 150 mg
C ❏ 5 mg
D ❏ 10 mg
E ❏ 200 mg

Select, from A to E, a strength in which the following products are available:

Q45   Dulco-lax tablets

Q46   Zantac tablets

Q47   Phenergan tablets

Q48   Imodium capsules

Questions 49–52 concern the following drugs:

A   ❑ norfloxacin
B   ❑ nicorandil
C   ❑ nifedipine
D   ❑ nitrofurantoin
E   ❑ naloxone

Select, from A to E, which one of the above corresponds to the drug brand name:

Q49   Macrodantin

Q50   Utinor

Q51   Ikorel

Q52   Adalat

Questions 53–83

Directions: For each of the questions below, ONE or MORE of the responses is (are) correct. Decide which of the responses is (are) correct. Then choose:

A   ❑ if 1, 2 and 3 are correct
B   ❑ if 1 and 2 only are correct
C   ❑ if 2 and 3 only are correct
D   ❑ if 1 only is correct
E   ❑ if 3 only is correct

Directions summarised				
A	B	C	D	E
1, 2, 3	1, 2 only	2, 3 only	1 only	3 only

Q53 When dispensing acarbose, the patient should be advised:

1   ❑ to take tablets in the morning
2   ❑ to avoid direct sunlight
3   ❑ that flatulence and diarrhoea may occur

Q54 Side-effects of esomeprazole include:

1   ❑ headache
2   ❑ pruritus
3   ❑ dizziness

Q55 Care should be taken with the use of the following drug(s) in older patients:

1   ❑ digoxin
2   ❑ trihexyphenidyl
3   ❑ lactulose

Q56 When dispensing mefloquine as a prophylaxis against malaria, the patient should be advised that:

1   ❑ tablets should be taken regularly
2   ❑ mosquito bites should be avoided
3   ❑ dizziness may occur as a side-effect

Q57   Symptoms of venous thrombosis include:

1   ❏ oedema
2   ❏ lower leg becoming bluish in colour
3   ❏ dry skin

Q58   In diabetes, blood glucose monitoring by the patient is of benefit:

1   ❏ to detect hypoglycaemia
2   ❏ to observe fluctuations in blood glucose over 24 hours
3   ❏ to make daily adjustments to insulin dose

Q59   Carcinoma of the large bowel could present:

1   ❏ with symptoms of bowel obstruction
2   ❏ at an advanced stage
3   ❏ with melaena

Q60   Clinical signs of tuberculosis include:

1   ❏ persistent cough
2   ❏ fever
3   ❏ weight loss

Q61   Diagnosis of head lice infestation is based on:

1   ❏ detection combing
2   ❏ hair cleanliness
3   ❏ hair texture

Q62   Which of the symptoms are characteristic of acute bronchitis?

1   ❏ chest tightness
2   ❏ purulent sputum
3   ❏ wheeziness

Q63   Symptoms of tinea pedis include:

1   ❑ itchiness
2   ❑ location mostly in interdigital space
3   ❑ white, macerated skin

Q64   Interferon beta:

1   ❑ can be administered orally and parenterally
2   ❑ may cause myalgia and fever
3   ❑ is used in multiple sclerosis

Q65   Tamoxifen:

1   ❑ is an oestrogen receptor agonist
2   ❑ presents a risk of endometrial cancer
3   ❑ is used in breast cancer in post-menopausal women with metastatic disease

Q66   Bromocriptine should be used with caution in:

1   ❑ renal impairment
2   ❑ schizophrenia
3   ❑ pregnancy

Q67   Which of the following cytotoxic drugs can be administered orally?

1   ❑ capecitabine
2   ❑ cyclophosphamide
3   ❑ carboplatin

Q68   Dydrogesterone:

1   ❑ is a progesterone analogue
2   ❑ is indicated for endometriosis
3   ❑ is contraindicated in severe liver impairment

Q69 Which of the products could be used to counteract the vasomotor symptoms associated with menopause?

1 ❑ Premarin
2 ❑ Livial
3 ❑ Yasmin

Q70 Side-effects associated with testosterone include:

1 ❑ headache
2 ❑ hirsutism
3 ❑ gynaecomastia

Q71 Levofloxacin:

1 ❑ has greater activity against pneumococci than ciprofloxacin
2 ❑ should be used with caution in patients with a history of epilepsy
3 ❑ may cause tremor and tachycardia

Q72 A patient presents at the pharmacy with a lesion, which appears to be a hard plaque with a central black area, on the underside of the foot:

1 ❑ patient should be referred immediately
2 ❑ patient should be asked about medical history of diabetes
3 ❑ products containing salicylic acid can be recommended

Q73 Lichen planus:

1 ❑ may involve gingival tissue
2 ❑ treatment may involve corticosteroids
3 ❑ pruritus occurs in most cases

Q74   Chickenpox:

1   ❑ is caused by herpes simplex
2   ❑ could be contracted from contact with a patient with shingles
3   ❑ promethazine could be used

Q75   Terbinafine:

1   ❑ may be administered orally in onychomycosis
2   ❑ could cause photosensitivity
3   ❑ treatment should not exceed 2 weeks

Q76   For anti-lice lotions:

1   ❑ alcoholic formulations are more effective
2   ❑ alcoholic formulations should be avoided in asthmatic patients
3   ❑ routine use is recommended as a prophylaxis

Q77   Rosiglitazone:

1   ❑ is a biguanide
2   ❑ should not be used with gliclazide
3   ❑ should be used with caution in patients with cardiovascular disease

Q78   Compared with soluble insulin, insulin aspart:

1   ❑ has a faster onset of action
2   ❑ results in a higher fasting blood-glucose concentration
3   ❑ is associated with a lower frequency of hypoglycaemia

Q79   Fluconazole:

1   ❑ may be used in vaginal candidiasis
2   ❑ is a triazole antifungal
3   ❑ when administered concomitantly with glibenclamide results in a lower plasma concentration of glibenclamide

Q80   Which of the following statements about cradle cap is (are) true?

1   ❑ it is a form of seborrhoeic dermatitis
2   ❑ baby oil could be used to relieve the condition
3   ❑ it is contagious

Q81   Examples of non-steroidal anti-inflammatory products include:

1   ❑ Oruvail
2   ❑ Feldene
3   ❑ Nootropil

Q82   For which of the following infections is antibacterial treatment NOT usually recommended:

1   ❑ typhoid fever
2   ❑ impetigo
3   ❑ gastroenteritis

Q83   The following is (are) effective in the management of nappy rash:

1   ❑ zinc and castor oil ointment
2   ❑ mepyramine cream
3   ❑ Eurax cream

Questions 84–88

Directions: The following questions consist of a first statement followed by a second statement. Decide whether the first statement is true or false. Decide whether the second statement is true or false. Then choose:

A   ❑ if both statements are true and the second statement is a *correct explanation* of the first statement

B   ❑ if both statements are true but the second statement *is NOT a correct explanation* of the first statement

C   ❑ if the first statement is true but the second statement is false

D   ❑ if the first statement is false but the second statement is true

E   ❑ if both statements are false

Directions summarised			
	First statement	**Second statement**	
A	True	True	Second statement is a *correct explanation* of the first
B	True	True	Second statement is *NOT a correct explanation* of the first
C	True	False	
D	False	True	
E	False	False	

Q84   Paclitaxel is a cytotoxic antibiotic. Paclitaxel is used in primary ovarian cancer.

Q85   The combination of antibacterial agents in co-trimoxazole presents a synergistic activity. Co-trimoxazole is associated with rare but serious side-effects.

Q86   Pethidine is a less potent analgesic than morphine. Pethidine is not suitable for severe, continuous pain.

Q87   All tetracyclines are effective against *Neisseria meningitidis*. Tetracyclines are used in acne.

Q88   Zafirlukast is a leukotriene-receptor antagonist. Zafirlukast is used in the treatment of an acute severe asthma attack.

Questions 89–100

Directions: These questions involve cases. Read the prescription or case and answer the questions.

Questions 89–90: Use the prescription below

Patient's name: . . . .

Xenical capsules
1 caps b.d. p.c.   m. 30

Doctor's signature: . . . .

Q89   In which condition is the product used?

A   ❑ anorexia
B   ❑ asthenia
C   ❑ obesity
D   ❑ bulimia
E   ❑ cholestasis

Q90   Xenical

1   ❑ is a pancreatic lipase inhibitor
2   ❑ may cause faecal urgency
3   ❑ may be administered twice daily

A   ❑ 1, 2, 3
B   ❑ 1, 2 only
C   ❑ 2, 3 only
D   ❑ 1 only
E   ❑ 3 only

Questions 91–94: Use the prescription below

Patient's name: . . . .

Daktacort cream
b.d. for 1 week   m. 1 tube

Doctor's signature: . . . .

Q91   The active ingredient(s) of Daktacort is (are):

A   ❑ econazole
B   ❑ hydrocortisone
C   ❑ econazole, hydrocortisone
D   ❑ miconazole, hydrocortisone
E   ❑ miconazole

Q92   Daktacort

1   ❑ is rarely associated with side-effects
2   ❑ should be discarded 5 days after opening
3   ❑ is also available as powder

A   ❑ 1, 2, 3
B   ❑ 1, 2 only
C   ❑ 2, 3 only
D   ❑ 1 only
E   ❑ 3 only

Q93   Daktacort is prescribed when the patient has:

A   ❑ fungal infection
B   ❑ dry skin
C   ❑ bacterial infection
D   ❑ acne
E   ❑ psoriasis

Q94   The pharmacist should advise the patient to apply Daktacort

1   ❏ sparingly
2   ❏ three times daily
3   ❏ for 6 months

A   ❏ 1, 2, 3
B   ❏ 1, 2 only
C   ❏ 2, 3 only
D   ❏ 1 only
E   ❏ 3 only

Questions 95–100: Use the patient profile below

```
Patient medication profile

Patient's name:        . . . . . . . . . . . . . . . . . . . . . . .

Age: 42 years
Allergies: none
Diagnosis: peptic ulcer disease, hypertension
Prescribed medication:   amoxicillin 1 g b.d.
                         omeprazole 20 mg b.d.
                         clarithromycin 500 mg b.d.
```

Q95   The duration of treatment that has been prescribed is usually:

A   ❏ 7 days
B   ❏ 3 days
C   ❏ 30 days
D   ❏ 5 days
E   ❏ 10 days

Q96   The pharmacist should advise the patient against the use of:

1   ❏ Nurofen
2   ❏ Clarityn
3   ❏ Rennie

A	❑	1, 2, 3
B	❑	1, 2 only
C	❑	2, 3 only
D	❑	1 only
E	❑	3 only

Q97 Adverse effects that could be experienced by the patient include:

1	❑	diarrhoea
2	❑	headache
3	❑	dry mouth

A	❑	1, 2, 3
B	❑	1, 2 only
C	❑	2, 3 only
D	❑	1 only
E	❑	3 only

Q98 Which is the preferred proprietary product that could be dispensed for clarithromycin?

A	❑	Klaricid
B	❑	Orelox
C	❑	Zithromax
D	❑	Erythroped
E	❑	Ketek

Q99 Losec MUPS:

1	❑	contains omeprazole
2	❑	could be dispersed in water or fruit juice
3	❑	could be chewed

A	❑	1, 2, 3
B	❑	1, 2 only
C	❑	2, 3 only
D	❑	1 only
E	❑	3 only

Q100 Prior to prescribing this treatment, which conditions should be excluded?

1 ❑ breast-feeding
2 ❑ gastric carcinoma
3 ❑ *Helicobacter pylori* infection

A ❑ 1, 2, 3
B ❑ 1, 2 only
C ❑ 2, 3 only
D ❑ 1 only
E ❑ 3 only

Test 1

Answers

A1   C

Fucicort contains fusidic acid (antibacterial) and betamethasone (corticosteroid), which is more potent than hydrocortisone (corticosteroid). Fucidin H contains fusidic acid and hydrocortisone; Daktacort contains miconazole (imidazole antifungal) and hydrocortisone; Canesten HC contains clotrimazole (imidazole antifungal) and hydrocortisone. Otosporin contains hydrocortisone in combination with two antibacterial agents, namely neomycin and polymyxin.

A2   E

Headache accompanied by loss of consciousness, neck stiffness and neurological signs such as paraesthesia and slurred speech requires referral.

A3   B

Nifedipine is a calcium-channel blocker of the dihydropyridine group. It relaxes smooth muscle and dilates both coronary and peripheral arteries by interfering with the inward displacement of calcium-channel ions through the active cell membrane. Unlike verapamil, nifedipine can be given with beta-blockers. Long-acting formulations of nifedipine are preferred in the long-term treatment of hypertension.

A4   C

In response to the presence of antigenic stimuli, in seasonal allergic rhinitis (hay fever), mast cells and basophils are sensitised and inflammatory mediators, such as leukotrienes and prostaglandins, are released. Osteocytes are bone cells involved in bone formation.

A5   D

Information required in patient medication records includes name, age and gender of the patient, diagnosis, current medication therapies, and medication allergies.

A6   B

Uniflu contains paracetamol (non-opioid analgesic), codeine (opioid analgesic), caffeine, diphenydramine (antihistamine), phenylephrine (nasal decongestant) and ascorbic acid. Day Nurse is the closest equivalent to Uniflu, as it contains paracetamol, phenylpropanolamine (nasal decongestant) and dextromethorphan (antitussive). Actifed contains triprolidine (antihistamine) and pseudoephedrine (nasal decongestant). Phenergan and Xyzal contain the antihistamines promethazine and levocetirizine respectively, whereas Ventolin contains salbutamol, which is a bronchodilator (selective beta$_2$–adrenoceptor agonist).

A7   A

Odourless vaginal discharge is a common symptom of vaginal candidiasis. Vaginal candidiasis accompanied by abdominal pain and fever warrants referral. Vaginal candidiasis occurring in diabetic patients and during pregnancy indicates need for referral.

A8   D

Long-term use of stimulant laxatives, such as bisacodyl and senna, precipitates atonic non-functioning colon. In the elderly, constipation generally requires long-term management. Use of magnesium salts as laxatives is indicated when rapid evacuation is required. Long-term use of magnesium salts and liquid paraffin is not recommended. Lactulose is a semi-synthetic disaccharide, which can be given on a regular basis to elderly patients as a laxative preparation.

A9   A

Hydralazine is a vasodilator antihypertensive drug. Valsartan and losartan are specific angiotensin-II receptor antagonists; perindopril and lisinopril are angiotensin-converting enzyme inhibitors, thereby inhibiting the conversion of angiotensin-I into the more potent vasoconstrictor angiotensin-II.

A10   A

Concurrent administration of lithium and selective serotonin re-uptake inhibitors, such as paroxetine, results in an increased risk of central nervous system effects and lithium toxicity has been reported.

A11   A

Celecoxib, a non-steroidal anti-inflammatory drug, is a cyclo-oxygenase-2 selective inhibitor that is as effective as diclofenac and naproxen. It should be used for the shortest period required to control symptoms. Use is associated with an increased risk of thrombotic events and the cyclo-oxygenase-2 selective inhibitors are contraindicated in cerebrovascular disease. Mobic is the proprietary preparation of meloxicam.

A12   D

Theophylline is a drug with a narrow therapeutic index, plasma concentrations of which must be maintained at 10–20 mg/L. Plasma concentrations above 20 mg/L increase the severity and frequency of adverse effects.

A13   D

Motilium contains domperidone, which is a dopamine antagonist and acts on the chemoreceptor trigger zone. It is ineffective in motion sickness. Stugeron contains cinnarizine; Avomine and Phenergan contain promethazine; and Kwells contains hyoscine hydrobromide. Cinnarizine and promethazine are antihistamines, which are indicated in motion sickness and hyoscine hydrobromide is an antimuscarinic agent that is also used in motion sickness.

A14   E

Alfuzosin is a selective alpha-blocker, which relaxes smooth muscle, thereby increasing urinary flow rate. Because of its alpha-blockade effect, alfuzosin tends to lower the blood pressure and the first dose of the drug may lead to a hypotensive effect.

A15   D

Mupirocin is only available as cream or ointment intended for topical use.

A16   B

Diazepam is a prescription-only medicine whereas pethidine, morphine, alfentanil and remifentanil are controlled drugs.

A17   C

Famciclovir, which is the pro-drug of penciclovir, is indicated in acute genital herpes simplex and in the treatment of varicella zoster. Famciclovir is available as tablets. Valaciclovir is the ester of aciclovir.

A18   D

Herpes labialis or cold sores can be precipitated by trauma to the lips and sunlight. In patients whose immune system is compromised, such as in immunosuppression or in cases of viral infections, herpes labialis may be precipitated. Dental caries do not precipitate cold sores.

A19   A

Gardasil is a quadrivalent vaccine of the human papilloma virus (type 6, 11, 16, 18). It is used for the prevention of cervical cancer and other pre-cancerous lesions. It should be given early in a female's sexual life and it is licensed for use in females between 9 and 26 years of age. Administration is by intramuscular injection and three doses are required. Because the vaccine does not protect against all the strains of the virus, cervical screening is still required. Duration of protection after a complete course is still not established but it is suggested that protection is maintained for at least 6 years.

A20   D

Cilest contains ethinylestradiol and norgestimate whereas Yasmin contains ethinylestradiol in combination with drospirenone. Both are combined oral contraceptives available as tablets, which have to be taken once daily for 21 days. Both are contraindicated in patients with venous thromboembolic diseases.

A21   C

Hydrocortisone cream is indicated for the treatment of contact dermatitis. It is applied sparingly once or twice daily for a maximum period of 1 week. Eurax (crotamiton) is an antipruritic agent but it is of uncertain value. Sedating systemic antihistamines may help but Clarityn tablets would not be the treatment of choice as they contain loratadine, which is non-sedating. Preparations containing antifungals such as Pevaryl (econazole) and Canesten HC (clotrimazole, hydrocortisone) are of no use in the treatment of contact dermatitis.

A22   D

Buspar containing buspirone is indicated in short-term anxiety. Diazepam, Stilnoct containing zolpidem, Heminevrin containing clomethiazole, and Phenergan containing promethazine are all indicated in insomnia.

A23   C

Rhinocort Aqua and Nasonex are preparations containing topical nasal corticosteroids (budesonide and mometasone furoate respectively). Otrivine contains a nasal decongestant (xylometazoline) and Sudafed is a systemic preparation containing a nasal decongestant (phenylephrine). Molcer is a preparation for ear-wax removal and which contains docusate sodium. Emadine contains an antihistamine (emedastine) and is presented as eye drops.

A24   B

Bupivacaine is an anaesthetic with a slow onset but a long duration of action. It is indicated for continuous epidural analgesia in labour. Xylocaine is the proprietary preparation of lidocaine (lignocaine). Lidocaine injections are used in dentistry.

A25   D

Haloperidol is indicated for schizophrenia, severe anxiety, motor tics and intractable hiccup. It is not indicated in the treatment of parkinsonism, which may be aggravated through its use, as haloperidol tends to cause extrapyramidal symptoms.

A26   A

Twinrix is a vaccine combining hepatitis A virus units and hepatitis B surface antigen, thereby protecting against hepatitis A and B.

A27   B

Rotarix consists of live, attenuated rotavirus strains presented as powder for reconstitution intended for oral administration.

A28   D

Fluarix is an influenza vaccine containing the H and N component of the prevalent influenza strains, against which vaccination is recommended each year by the World Health Organization.

A29   B

Constipation is a side-effect of Zofran, which contains ondansetron.

A30   C

Cytotec containing misoprostol (prostaglandin analogue) may cause abnormal vaginal bleeding.

A31 E

Diamox containing acetazolamide (carbonic anhydrase inhibitor) may cause paraesthesia.

A32 E

Aldactone containing spironolactone (potassium-sparing diuretic and an aldosterone antagonist) is used with caution in cases of porphyria.

A33 B

Inderal containing propranolol (beta-adrenoceptor blocking agent) is used with caution in diabetic patients.

A34 B

Inderal containing propranolol (beta-adrenoceptor blocking agent) is used with caution in myasthenia gravis.

A35 D

Byetta containing exenatide (incretin mimetic) is marketed by Lilly.

A36 A

Nexium containing esomeprazole (proton pump inhibitor) is marketed by AstraZeneca.

A37 C

Alupent containing orciprenaline (non-selective $beta_2$–agonist bronchodilator) is marketed by Boehringer Ingelheim.

A38 C

Difflam containing benzydamine (local analgesic) is available as an oral rinse and is indicated for inflammatory conditions of the oropharynx and for palliative relief in post-radiation mucositis.

A39 B

Rynacrom containing sodium cromoglicate is available as a nasal spray used in allergic rhinitis.

A40 D

Molcer ear drops containing sodium docusate is a preparation used to remove ear wax.

A41 C

Liver function tests must be carried out before and within 1–3 months of starting treatment with statins, such as fluvastatin. Liver function tests are thereafter carried out at 6-month intervals for 1 year.

A42 E

Selective serotonin re-uptake inhibitors, such as fluvoxamine, are used with caution in patients with epilepsy and should be discontinued if convulsions occur.

A43 D

Lithium therapy necessitates the monitoring of thyroid function every 6–12 months in stabilised patients. Occurrence of symptoms such as lethargy, which may reflect hypothyroidism, should be monitored.

A44 A

Levodopa must be used with caution in patients suffering from endocrine disorders such as diabetes mellitus.

A45 C

Dulco-lax containing bisacodyl (stimulant laxative) is available as 5 mg tablets.

A46   B

Zantac containing ranitidine (H_2-receptor antagonist) is available as 75 mg, 150 mg or 300 mg tablets.

A47   D

Phenergan, containing promethazine (sedating antihistamine), is available as 10 mg or 25 mg tablets.

A48   A

Imodium containing loperamide (antidiarrhoeal) is available as 2 mg capsules.

A49   D

Macrodantin is a proprietary preparation of nitrofurantoin, an anti-infective agent used in urinary tract infections.

A50   A

Utinor is a proprietary preparation of norfloxacin (quinolone).

A51   B

Ikorel is a proprietary preparation of nicorandil (an anti-anginal drug).

A52   C

Adalat is a proprietary preparation of nifedipine (a dihydropyridine calcium-channel blocker).

A53   E

Acarbose, an antidiabetic that inhibits intestinal alpha glucosidases, may cause flatulence and diarrhoea. The tablets, which can be taken three times daily, must be taken before food.

A54   A

Esomeprazole is a proton pump inhibitor and may cause headache, pruritus and dizziness as side-effects.

A55   B

Digoxin (cardiac glycoside) and trihexyphenidyl (antimuscarinic drug) must be used with caution in elderly patients. Low doses are recommended in elderly patients to avoid toxicity. Lactulose may be safely administered to elderly patients with constipation.

A56   A

Patients taking mefloquine as prophylaxis against malaria should be advised to take the medication regularly and to avoid mosquito bites. Dizziness may be caused by mefloquine and patients should be informed about this side-effect.

A57   B

Venous thrombosis results in congestion in the affected foot. The foot becomes painful, swollen and blue or black in colour, caused by lack of blood circulation.

A58   B

Blood glucose monitoring measures the concentration at the time of the test. Monitoring in diabetic patients is essential to detect fluctuations in blood glucose concentrations and to help detect hypoglycaemia. Patients should be trained and encouraged to measure their blood glucose concentrations regularly. This would allow for alterations of their insulin dose made once or twice weekly. It is not recommended to alter the insulin dose on a daily basis, except during illness when patients are under medical supervision.

A59   A

Cancer of the large bowel can present with symptoms of bowel obstruction, such as nausea, vomiting, colicky pain, constipation and abdominal distension. Blood in the stools (melaena) is a classic symptom of colorectal cancer. Cancer of the large bowel may be at an advanced stage before the symptoms are present.

A60   A

Symptoms of tuberculosis, which are mild in the early stages of the disease, include persistent cough, fever and weight loss.

A61   D

Detection of head lice infestation is based on identifying lice by detection combing. Head lice detection cannot be solely based on an itchy scalp because not all children with head lice have the symptom. Furthermore, itchiness is caused by an allergic reaction to the lice, which may develop a few weeks after the infection and can persist for some time after eradication. Infestation is equally likely to occur in clean or dirty hair.

A62   A

Symptoms characteristic of acute bronchitis include chest tightness, cough with purulent sputum, chest soreness, wheeziness, and difficulty in breathing.

A63   A

Tinea pedis or athelete's foot is a fungal infection affecting the feet, classically starting between the fourth and fifth toes but which can spread to other areas of the foot. The classic symptoms include itchiness and redness in the affected area, which later on becomes white, macerated and sore.

A64   C

Interferon beta, which is indicated for multiple sclerosis, is administered parenterally only. The most common side-effects are irritation at the injection site and influenza-like symptoms, such as fever, myalgia, chills and malaise. The side-effects tend to decrease with time.

A65 C

Tamoxifen is an oestrogen-receptor antagonist. It is used in post-menopausal women with oestrogen-receptor-positive metastatic breast cancer at a dose of 20 mg daily. It can also be used in combination with chemotherapy. Severe side-effects are infrequent; however, it is associated with a small risk of endometrial cancer. Patients should be informed and reassured that the benefits of the treatment at this dose outweigh the risk.

A66 C

Administration of bromocriptine necessitates monitoring pituitary gland function, especially during pregnancy, whereas in psychotic disorders, including schizophrenia, bromocriptine must be administered with caution. There is no need to reduce the dose or administer bromocriptine with caution in patients with renal impairment.

A67 B

Capecitabine is an antimetabolite neoplastic and cyclophosphamide is an alkylating neoplastic, both of which can be administered orally. Carboplatin is a platinum compound (antineoplastic). All currently available platinum compounds are administered parenterally via the intravenous route.

A68 A

Dydrogesterone is a progesterone analogue. One of its indications is endometriosis, in which case dydrogesterone is administered at a dose of 10 mg two to three times daily. Progestogens are contraindicated in severe liver impairment and in patients with a history of liver tumours.

A69 B

Premarin is a preparation containing conjugated oestrogens indicated to relieve vasomotor symptoms in menopause for women who have undergone hysterectomy. Livial is a preparation containing tibolone. Tibolone combines oestrogenic, progestogenic and weak androgenic activity and helps relieve vasomotor symptoms associated with menopause. Yasmin is a combined oral contraceptive containing ethinylestradiol and drospirenone and is not indicated in menopause.

A70 A

Side-effects associated with testosterone include headache, hirsutism and gynaecomastia.

A71 A

Both levofloxacin and ciprofloxacin are quinolones active against both Gram-negative and Gram-positive bacteria. However, levofloxacin has greater activity against pneumoccocci than ciprofloxacin. Levofloxacin may cause tremor and tachycardia as side-effects. All quinolones should be administered with caution in patients with a history of epilepsy.

A72 C

The description given is typical of verrucas. Verrucas are plantar warts caused by the human papilloma virus affecting the sole of the foot in pressure areas. The lesion is pushed into the epidermis eventually forming a dry hard plaque with a small central black core, which comprises blood vessels. Preparations containing salicylic acid, which is a keratolytic agent, may be used as treatment. Diabetic patients should be referred.

A73 A

Lichen planus is a condition of unknown aetiology presenting as small pruritic and shiny papules, which initially may appear purple in colour. It affects the limbs, wrists, trunk, genitalia and the mouth, in which case ulcerated lesions occur on the gingival tissue. Treatment for lichen planus involves the use of systemic antihistamines but sometimes corticosteroids are required.

A74 C

Chickenpox is caused by the virus herpes zoster, which could be contracted from patients with shingles but not vice versa. Calamine lotion or oral sedative antihistamines, such as promethazine, are used to provide relief from the itchy vesicles typical of chickenpox.

A75 B

Terbinafine is available for oral administration and is indicated for fungal nail infections. Treatment with terbinafine for nail infections can take up to 3 months depending on the condition, with a minimum duration of 6 weeks. Photosensitivity may occur as a side-effect to terbinafine.

A76 B

Anti-lice alcoholic preparations are considered more effective than aqueous preparations. However, alcoholic preparations are unsuitable for use in children and patients with asthma and eczema. Anti-lice preparations should not be used for prophylaxis because they are ineffective and may encourage the development of resistance.

A77 E

Rosiglitazone is a thiazolidinedione that can be used in combination with metformin or a sulphonylurea such as gliclazide. Rosiglitazone should be administered with caution in patients with cardiovascular disease.

A78 A

When compared with soluble insulin, the human analogue insulin aspart has a faster onset and a shorter duration of action, resulting in a higher fasting and preprandial blood glucose concentration. The incidence of hypoglycaemia tends to be lower with insulin aspart than with soluble insulin.

A79 B

Fluconazole is a triazole antifungal that may be administered in recurrent vaginal candidiasis. Fluconazole interacts with sulphonylureas such as glibenclamide, resulting in increased plasma concentrations of the sulphonylurea.

A80 B

Cradle cap is a form of seborrhoeic dermatitis of the scalp affecting babies aged 1–3 months. The condition is not contagious and can be treated by rubbing baby oil into the scalp, leaving it overnight and shampooing afterwards.

A81 B

Oruvail is a proprietary preparation of ketoprofen and Feldene is a proprietary preparation of piroxicam, both of which are non-steroidal anti-inflammatory drugs; Nootropil is a proprietary preparation of piracetam, which is not a non-steroidal anti-inflammatory drug. Nootropil is indicated as adjunctival treatment in cortical myoclonus.

A82 E

Antibacterial treatment is generally not required in cases of gastroenteritis. Typhoid fever is treated with ciprofloxacin (quinolone), cefotaxime (third generation cephalosporin) or chloramphenicol. Impetigo necessitates the systemic use of flucloxacillin or erythromycin. Topical fusidic acid or mupirocin may also be used.

A83 D

Nappy rash is effectively managed by the application of a barrier preparation, such as zinc and castor oil ointment. Antihistamine creams such as mepyramine and antipruritic creams such as Eurax cream, containing crotamiton, are of no use.

A84 D

Paclitaxel is a taxane antineoplastic used in the treatment of primary ovarian cancer.

A85 B

Co-trimoxazole refers to the combination of sulfamethoxazole and trimethoprim, which offers synergistic activity. Co-trimoxazole is associated with rare but serious side-effects, such as Stevens-Johnson syndrome, bone marrow suppression and blood dyscrasias.

A86   B

Pethidine is a less potent opioid analgesic than morphine. Pethidine is not suitable for continuous pain because of its short-lasting analgesia.

A87   D

Minocycline differs from the other tetracyclines in that it is active against *Neisseria meningitidis*. Topical and systemic preparations of tetracyclines are indicated in acne.

A88   C

Zafirlukast is a leukotriene-receptor antagonist. Leukotriene-receptor antagonists are used for prophylaxis of asthma and should not be used to relieve an attack of acute severe asthma.

A89   C

Xenical is a proprietary preparation of orlistat, which is used as an adjunct to diet in the treatment of obesity.

A90   A

The active ingredient of Xenical, orlistat, is a pancreatic lipase inhibitor. Side-effects include faecal urgency, liquid oily stools and flatulence. Xenical capsules are administered before, during or up to 1 hour after the two main meals, twice daily.

A91   D

Daktacort cream is a trade name for a preparation containing miconazole (imidazole antifungal) and hydrocortisone (corticosteroid).

A92 D

As Daktacort cream contains hydrocortisone, a mild steroid, its use is rarely associated with side-effects unlike the potent and very potent steroids. The product is generally applied once or twice daily for 1 week. It should be discarded once the expiry date has elapsed. Daktacort is only available as cream or ointment.

A93 A

Daktacort preparations are indicated when patients have fungal infections accompanied by inflammation of the skin.

A94 D

In this case Daktacort cream should be applied sparingly, twice daily for 1 week.

A95 A

The therapy prescribed is a 1-week triple therapy regimen consisting of amoxicillin, clarithromycin and omeprazole against *Helicobacter pylori* infection.

A96 D

Nurofen is a proprietary preparation of ibuprofen, a non-steroidal anti-inflammatory drug which, as a side-effect, may cause peptic ulceration. Nurofen is contraindicated in patients with active ulceration and the patient is being treated for peptic ulceration. Therefore Nurofen should not be used. Clarityn, which contains the non-sedating antihistamine loratadine; and Rennie, which is an antacid containing calcium carbonate and magnesium carbonate, do not cause gastrointestinal bleeding and may be taken by the patient.

A97 A

Headache, diarrhoea and dry mouth are side-effects that may be caused by omeprazole.

A98   A

Klaricid is a proprietary preparation of clarithromycin. Orelox is a proprietary preparation of cefpodoxime; Zithromax contains azithromycin; Erythroped contains erythromycin; and Ketek contains telithromycin.

A99   B

Losec MUPS is a proprietary preparation of omeprazole available as dispersible tablets that can be dispersed either in water or fruit juice. Tablets should not be chewed.

A100   B

Proton pump inhibitors such as omeprazole may mask the symptoms of gastric cancer. Omeprazole is best avoided during breast-feeding. The prescription is indicative of triple therapy used as eradication therapy in *H. pylori* infection.

Test 2

Questions

Questions 1–21

Directions: Each of the questions or incomplete statements is followed by five suggested answers. Select the best answer in each case.

Q1   All of the following products contain aspirin EXCEPT:

A   ❑ Syndol
B   ❑ Alka-Seltzer
C   ❑ Anadin Extra
D   ❑ Nu-Seals
E   ❑ Aspro

Q2   The management of unstable angina includes all EXCEPT:

A   ❑ aspirin
B   ❑ exercise stress test
C   ❑ clopidogrel
D   ❑ isosorbide dinitrate
E   ❑ atenolol

Q3   Digoxin:

A   ❑ clearance is by the liver
B   ❑ increases conduction of the AV node
C   ❑ decreases the force of myocardial contraction
D   ❑ has a short half-life
E   ❑ may cause atrial tachycardia in overdosage

Q4 Which of the following causes bronchodilatation?

A ❑ adrenaline (epinephrine)
B ❑ histamine
C ❑ prostaglandin E2
D ❑ kinins
E ❑ guaifenesin

Q5 Information sources recommended to be available in a dispensary include all EXCEPT:

A ❑ *British National Formulary*
B ❑ *Gray's Anatomy*
C ❑ *Martindale: The Complete Drug Reference*
D ❑ pharmacy legislation
E ❑ *Pharmacological Basis of Therapeutics*

Q6 What is an appropriate therapeutic alternative for Clarinase?

A ❑ Cirrus
B ❑ Actifed
C ❑ Xyzal
D ❑ Clarityn
E ❑ Telfast

Q7 A patient who is infested with *Enterobius vermicularis* probably has:

A ❑ duodenal haemorrhaging
B ❑ increased urinary output
C ❑ nocturnal perianal pruritus
D ❑ diarrhoea
E ❑ abdominal pain

Q8   A patient asks for an over-the-counter cold remedy. The pharmacist could appropriately suggest:

A   ❑ Otrivine drops
B   ❑ Beecham's Hot Lemon and Honey powders
C   ❑ Atarax tablets
D   ❑ Actifed Compound Linctus
E   ❑ Karvol inhalation capsules

Q9   Which of the following drugs acts by enzyme inhibition?

A   ❑ salbutamol
B   ❑ acetazolamide
C   ❑ tolbutamide
D   ❑ chlorpromazine
E   ❑ zafirlukast

Q10   A significant clinical interaction may occur if sildenafil is administered concomitantly with:

A   ❑ Zantac tablets
B   ❑ Tagamet tablets
C   ❑ Isordil tablets
D   ❑ Augmentin tablets
E   ❑ Tenormin tablets

Q11   Famciclovir can be used in the treatment of:

A   ❑ chickenpox
B   ❑ influenza
C   ❑ warts
D   ❑ rubella
E   ❑ mumps

Q12   Ergotamine is used as an antimigraine drug because it:

   A   ❏ is a beta-adrenergic agonist
   B   ❏ causes vasoconstriction
   C   ❏ inhibits platelet aggregation
   D   ❏ causes elevation of the pain threshold
   E   ❏ is a prostaglandin antagonist

Q13   For the intravenous administration of hydrocortisone, a suitable formulation is:

   A   ❏ base
   B   ❏ acetate
   C   ❏ propionate
   D   ❏ cypionate
   E   ❏ sodium succinate

Q14   The site of action of Lasilix is at the:

   A   ❏ distal tubule
   B   ❏ proximal tubule
   C   ❏ collecting duct
   D   ❏ loop of Henle
   E   ❏ glomerular membrane

Q15   All of the following skin disorders are worsened by sun exposure EXCEPT:

   A   ❏ seborrhoeic dermatitis
   B   ❏ furuncles
   C   ❏ chloasma
   D   ❏ acne vulgaris
   E   ❏ herpes simplex labialis

Q16 Drugs that are commercially available in more than one strength include all EXCEPT:

A   ❏ Flagyl tablets
B   ❏ Istin tablets
C   ❏ Risperdal tablets
D   ❏ Naprosyn capsules
E   ❏ Migril tablets

Q17 Triamcinolone differs from hydrocortisone in that it:

A   ❏ is less potent as an anti-inflammatory
B   ❏ is available in the oral dosage form
C   ❏ has a longer duration of action
D   ❏ has more mineralocorticoid activity
E   ❏ is available for topical application

Q18 What is the most appropriate treatment for a mycotic vaginal super-infection?

A   ❏ Betadine douche
B   ❏ Ortho-Gynest cream
C   ❏ Lamisil tablets
D   ❏ Gyno-Daktarin pessary
E   ❏ Canesten cream

Q19 Which of the following products is NOT indicated as an agent to be used in gastrointestinal ulcer healing?

A   ❏ omeprazole
B   ❏ rabeprazole
C   ❏ misoprostol
D   ❏ loperamide
E   ❏ ranitidine

Q20 Cradle cap:

A ❑ is a form of seborrhoeic dermatitis
B ❑ occurs in children over 1 year
C ❑ may be treated initially with corticosteroid scalp application
D ❑ is a lifelong condition
E ❑ is a form of food allergy

Q21 What class of drugs does the structure below represent?

A ❑ oestrogens
B ❑ phenothiazines
C ❑ non-steroidal anti-inflammatory drugs
D ❑ antidepressants
E ❑ glucocorticoids

Questions 22–48

Directions: Each group of questions below consists of five lettered headings followed by a list of numbered questions. For each numbered question select the one heading that is most closely related to it. Each heading may be used once, more than once, or not at all.

Questions 22–24 concern the following manufacturers:

A ❏ Bayer
B ❏ Novartis
C ❏ GlaxoSmithKline
D ❏ AstraZeneca
E ❏ Janssen-Cilag

Select, from A to E, which one of the above manufacturers is associated with the trademarked product:

Q22 Daktarin cream

Q23 Otrivine drops

Q24 Rhinocort Aqua

Questions 25–27 concern the following products:

A ❏ Buscopan
B ❏ Zaditen
C ❏ Voltarol
D ❏ Natrilix
E ❏ Lescol

Select, from A to E, the product that should be used with caution in each of the following conditions:

Q25 prostatic hypertrophy

Q26 asthma

Q27 gout

Questions 28–30 concern the following life-threatening adverse reactions:

    A   ❑ agranulocytosis
    B   ❑ pseudomembranous colitis
    C   ❑ respiratory depression
    D   ❑ cardiovascular collapse
    E   ❑ nephrotoxicity

Select, from A to E, the adverse reaction that may occur following administration of the following drugs:

Q28   acetazolamide

Q29   amoxicillin

Q30   atracurium

Questions 31–33 concern the following drugs:

    A   ❑ doxorubicin
    B   ❑ methotrexate
    C   ❑ mitomycin
    D   ❑ cyclophosphamide
    E   ❑ tamoxifen

Select, from A to E, which one of the above:

Q31   is limited in its clinical usefulness by cardiotoxicity

Q32   may be used in severe resistant psoriasis

Q33   has a mechanism of action involving alkylation

Questions 34–36 concern the following products:

A ❑ Suboxone
B ❑ Anadin Extra
C ❑ Cerumol
D ❑ Difflam
E ❑ Optrex

Select, from A to E, which one of the above:

Q34 has astringent properties

Q35 contains buprenorphine with naloxone

Q36 contains caffeine

Questions 37–40 concern the following drugs:

A ❑ sumatriptan
B ❑ ondansetron
C ❑ tramadol
D ❑ cyclizine
E ❑ pizotifen

Select, from A to E, which one of the above:

Q37 is used in the treatment of acute migraine

Q38 is an opioid analgesic

Q39 should not be used in ischaemic heart disease

Q40 is a specific serotonin antagonist

Questions 41–44 concern the following strengths:

A   ❏ 5%
B   ❏ 2%
C   ❏ 20%
D   ❏ 0.05%
E   ❏ 10%

Select, from A to E, a strength in which the following products are available:

Q41   aciclovir cream

Q42   mupirocin ointment

Q43   azelaic acid

Q44   fluticasone cream

Questions 45–48 concern the following drugs:

A   ❏ mebeverine
B   ❏ mebendazole
C   ❏ meloxicam
D   ❏ meprobamate
E   ❏ melatonin

Select, from A to E, which one of the above corresponds to the drug brand name:

Q45   Mobic

Q46   Vermox

Q47   Colofac

Q48   Circadin

Questions 49–79

Directions: For each of the questions below, ONE or MORE of the responses is (are) correct. Decide which of the responses is (are) correct. Then choose:

A   ❏ if 1, 2 and 3 are correct
B   ❏ if 1 and 2 only are correct
C   ❏ if 2 and 3 only are correct
D   ❏ if 1 only is correct
E   ❏ if 3 only is correct

Directions summarised				
A	**B**	**C**	**D**	**E**
1, 2, 3	1, 2 only	2, 3 only	1 only	3 only

Q49   When dispensing alfuzosin hydrochloride, the patient should be advised to:

1   ❏ take the first dose at night before retiring to bed
2   ❏ be careful when driving
3   ❏ avoid alcoholic drink

Q50   Side-effects of venlafaxine include:

1   ❏ diarrhoea
2   ❏ headache
3   ❏ blurred vision

Q51   Care should be taken with the use of the following drugs in a patient with renal impairment:

1   ❏ aciclovir
2   ❏ amoxicillin
3   ❏ naproxen

Q52   When dispensing phenytoin, the patient should be advised:

1   ❑ to keep taking the medicine routinely as directed
2   ❑ to report promptly symptoms of bruising or unexplained bleeding
3   ❑ that visual symptoms commonly occur

Q53   Symptoms of endometriosis include:

1   ❑ infertility
2   ❑ vaginal discharge
3   ❑ pelvic pain a few days after termination of menstruation

Q54   Which of the following vaccines are usually started before 6 months of age?

1   ❑ polio vaccine
2   ❑ pertussis vaccine
3   ❑ BCG vaccine

Q55   Gastro-oesophageal reflux in infants:

1   ❑ usually requires surgical intervention
2   ❑ is extremely rare
3   ❑ may be alleviated by thickening feeds

Q56   Clinical signs of dehydration in children include:

1   ❑ tachycardia
2   ❑ loss of skin turgor
3   ❑ dry tongue

Q57   Clinical features of mumps include:

1   ❑ enlargement of parotid glands
2   ❑ fever
3   ❑ bronchitis

Q58   Which symptoms are characteristic of allergic rhinitis?

1   ❏ shortness of breath
2   ❏ conjunctival lacrimation
3   ❏ prolonged sneezing attacks

Q59   Symptoms of cataracts include:

1   ❏ ocular pain
2   ❏ watery eyes
3   ❏ reduction in visual acuity

Q60   Calcipotriol:

1   ❏ may cause skin discoloration
2   ❏ is a vitamin D derivative
3   ❏ is used for psoriasis

Q61   Ciclosporin:

1   ❏ may cause nephrotoxicity
2   ❏ is associated with gastrointestinal disturbances
3   ❏ is only available as a parenteral preparation

Q62   Ciprofloxacin should be used with caution in:

1   ❏ epileptic patients
2   ❏ children
3   ❏ pregnancy

Q63   Which of the following drugs should be swallowed whole, not chewed?

1   ❏ Arthrotec tablets
2   ❏ Voltarol Retard tablets
3   ❏ Dulco-lax tablets

Q64   Ranitidine:

1   ❑ interferes significantly with concomitant warfarin therapy
2   ❑ has a maximum maintenance dose for reflux oesophagitis of
       150 mg at night
3   ❑ reduces gastric acid output

Q65   Which of the following drugs could cause nausea and vomiting as a
          side-effect?

1   ❑ prednisolone
2   ❑ omeprazole
3   ❑ paclitaxel

Q66   Side-effects associated with levodopa include:

1   ❑ insomnia
2   ❑ discoloration of urine
3   ❑ headache

Q67   The use of heparins for the management of thrombo-embolic disease
          in pregnancy:

1   ❑ is supported since they do not cross the placenta
2   ❑ should be stopped at onset of labour
3   ❑ may result in maternal osteoporosis

Q68   A patient presents at the pharmacy with a headache that is constantly
          painful and seems to be worse in the morning:

1   ❑ patient should be asked about a medical history of hyperten-
       sion
2   ❑ referral should be considered if episode is accompanied by
       fever, neck stiffness
3   ❑ the headache is characteristically tumorigenic

Q69   Periodontitis:

1   ❑ involves the peritoneum
2   ❑ requires referral
3   ❑ is an inflammatory condition

Q70   In cystitis:

1   ❑ the use of alkalinising agents as a treatment modality is associated with a clinically significant risk of hyperkalaemia
2   ❑ *Escherichia coli* is the most common cause
3   ❑ occurrence in children warrants referral

Q71   Tamoxifen:

1   ❑ is an oestrogen-receptor agonist
2   ❑ common side-effects expected include alopecia, uterine fibroids
3   ❑ is used as adjuvant hormonal treatment in breast cancer

Q72   Nicotine chewing gum in smoking cessation:

1   ❑ provides a residual nicotine level
2   ❑ requires one chewing gum for a minimum of 1 hour
3   ❑ may have aphthous ulceration as a side-effect

Q73   Zolpidem:

1   ❑ is a benzodiazepine
2   ❑ has a long duration of action
3   ❑ should be used with caution in patients with hepatic impairment

Q74   Orciprenaline:

1   ❑ is available only as a metered dose inhaler
2   ❑ is a selective beta2 adrenoceptor stimulant
3   ❑ can be prescribed for a child aged 4 years

Q75   Gliclazide:

1   ❏ when administered concomitantly with fluconazole, results in a lower plasma concentration of gliclazide
2   ❏ is a sulphonylurea
3   ❏ has a shorter half-life than glibenclamide

Q76   Which of the following statements about typhoid fever is (are) true?

1   ❏ it is caused by a coccus
2   ❏ it has an incubation period of 4 weeks
3   ❏ it may be associated with rose spots

Q77   Examples of antipsychotic drugs include:

1   ❏ Largactil
2   ❏ Serenace
3   ❏ Tegretol

Q78   For which of the following infections is prophylaxis undertaken by means of a vaccination programme?

1   ❏ hepatitis B
2   ❏ malaria
3   ❏ hepatitis C

Q79   The following are effective in the management of fungal nail infections:

1   ❏ griseofulvin
2   ❏ terbinafine
3   ❏ nystatin

Questions 80–88

Directions: The following questions consist of a first statement followed by a second statement. Decide whether the first statement is true or false. Decide whether the second statement is true or false. Then choose:

A   ❑ if both statements are true and the second statement is a *correct explanation* of the first statement

B   ❑ if both statements are true but the second statement *is NOT a correct explanation* of the first statement

C   ❑ if the first statement is true but the second statement is false

D   ❑ if the first statement is false but the second statement is true

E   ❑ if both statements are false

Directions summarised			
	First statement	**Second statement**	
A	True	True	Second statement is a *correct explanation* of the first
B	True	True	Second statement is *NOT a correct explanation* of the first
C	True	False	
D	False	True	
E	False	False	

Q80   Statins may be recommended to a 60-year-old asymptomatic male who is overweight, has a family history of coronary heart disease and is a smoker. The patient has a 10-year cardiovascular risk of 10% or more and is likely to benefit from statin treatment.

Q81   Ephedrine administered by slow intravenous injection may be used to reverse hypotension occurring after epidural anaesthesia. Ephedrine is a vasoconstrictor sympathomimetic agent, which should not be used in bradycardia.

Q82 Buccastem consists of prochlorperazine, a phenothiazine derivative, which is presented as tablets that are to be placed high between the upper lip and gum and allowed to dissolve there. It may be used in the treatment of nausea and vomiting associated with migraine, as absorption from the stomach, which is usually delayed in migraine, is avoided.

Q83 Flumazenil is a specific agonist used in anaesthesia to reverse the CNS depressant effects. Flumazenil should not be administered quickly to avoid too-rapid wakening, which could result in agitation, anxiety and fear.

Q84 Orlistat is an enzyme inhibitor. Orlistat should be taken three times daily.

Q85 Enalapril may precipitate a hypoglycaemic attack in a diabetic patient. Enalapril may potentiate the effect of sulphonylureas.

Q86 Repaglinide stimulates peripheral utilisation of glucose. Repaglinide is indicated only as monotherapy in diabetes mellitus.

Q87 Urinalysis for glucose monitoring is a good indicator of hypoglycaemia or hyperglycaemia. Blood glucose concentrations should be maintained at a constant level.

Q88 100 µg of budesonide are equivalent to 200 µg of fluticasone. Budesonide and fluticasone are both indicated for the prophylaxis of allergic rhinitis.

Questions 89–100

Directions: These questions involve cases. Read the prescription or case and answer the questions.

Questions 89–90: Use the prescription below

Patient's name: . . . .

Xalatan drops
1 drop o.n.   m. 1 bottle

Doctor's signature: . . . .

Q89   For which of these conditions are these eye drops prescribed?

A   ❑   cataracts
B   ❑   glaucoma
C   ❑   blepharitis
D   ❑   conjunctivitis
E   ❑   iritis

Q90   Xalatan:

1   ❑   is a prostaglandin analogue
2   ❑   may cause eye discoloration
3   ❑   is administered once daily

A   ❑   1, 2, 3
B   ❑   1, 2 only
C   ❑   2, 3 only
D   ❑   1 only
E   ❑   3 only

Questions 91–94:

A patient who is taking imipramine is diagnosed with hypertension.

For the following products, place your order of preference, assigning 1 to the product that should be recommended as first choice and 4 to the product that should be recommended as last choice.

Q91 bendroflumethiazide

Q92 furosemide

Q93 perindopril

Q94 propranolol

Questions 95–100: Use the patient profile below

Patient medication profile

Patient's name: . . . .

Age: 63 years
Allergies: none
Diagnosis: hypertension, arthritis, anxiety
Medication record: bendroflumethiazide tablets 2.5 mg daily
                   Zestril tablets 10 mg daily
                   Valium tablets 5 mg t.d.s.
                   Deltacortril tablets 10 mg daily
                   methotrexate tablets 2.5 mg as directed
                   paracetamol tablets 500 mg p.r.n.

Q95 Patients taking bendroflumethiazide are often given a potassium supplement. The patient may not need one because she is also taking:

A ❑ Valium
B ❑ Zestril
C ❑ Deltacortril
D ❑ methotrexate
E ❑ paracetamol

Q96   When dispensing the medications, the pharmacist should advise the patient against the concomitant use of:

1   ❑ Maalox
2   ❑ alcohol
3   ❑ Voltarol

A   ❑ 1, 2, 3
B   ❑ 1, 2 only
C   ❑ 2, 3 only
D   ❑ 1 only
E   ❑ 3 only

Q97   Patient should contact doctor if cough develops because:

1   ❑ methotrexate may cause pulmonary toxicity
2   ❑ it may indicate need of an antibacterial drug
3   ❑ it may indicate adrenal suppression

A   ❑ 1, 2, 3
B   ❑ 1, 2 only
C   ❑ 2, 3 only
D   ❑ 1 only
E   ❑ 3 only

Q98   Which of the following laboratory tests should be performed while the patient is taking methotrexate?

1   ❑ liver function tests
2   ❑ full blood count
3   ❑ renal function tests

A   ❑ 1, 2, 3
B   ❑ 1, 2 only
C   ❑ 2, 3 only
D   ❑ 1 only
E   ❑ 3 only

Q99   The patient is instructed to take methotrexate:

A ❑ daily
B ❑ twice daily
C ❑ every alternate day
D ❑ weekly
E ❑ monthly

Q100 Disadvantages of Deltacortril therapy include:

1 ❑ precipitation of osteoporosis
2 ❑ insomnia
3 ❑ candidiasis

A ❑ 1, 2, 3
B ❑ 1, 2 only
C ❑ 2, 3 only
D ❑ 1 only
E ❑ 3 only

Test 2

Answers

A1   A

Syndol is a combination analgesic containing paracetamol (non-opioid analgesic), codeine (opioid analgesic), caffeine and doxylamine (antihistamine). Alka-Seltzer is presented as effervescent tablets containing aspirin, citric acid and sodium bicarbonate. Anadin Extra is a combination analgesic containing aspirin, paracetamol and caffeine (a weak stimulant). Nu-Seals contains aspirin at the 75 mg dose per tablet. Aspro is an effervescent preparation of aspirin.

A2   B

Unstable angina is distinguished from stable angina by changes in frequency and severity of attacks. The aims of the management of angina are to provide supportive care and relief during an acute attack, and to prevent subsequent myocardial infarction and death. Patients should be admitted to hospital and drug therapy optimised. The management involves the administration of anti-platelet agents, namely aspirin and clopidogrel. Nitrates — for example, isosorbide dinitrate — are used to relieve ischaemic pain and act as vasodilators. Beta-blockers such as atenolol should be used in patients without contraindications. Patients are advised to avoid strenuous exercise (and therefore avoid undertaking the exercise stress test) to minimise the occurrence of attacks.

A3   E

Digoxin is a positive inotrope, hence it increases the force of myocardial contraction and may be effective in heart failure. It is a cardiac glycoside, which reduces the conductivity of the atrioventricular (AV) node and which may be used in atrial fibrillation. Digoxin has a long half-life and is given once daily. It is cleared by the renal system and hence renal impairment requires the reduction of digoxin dose. Arrhythmias, such as atrial tachycardia, may be a sign of digoxin toxicity. Digoxin toxicity is enhanced if there are electrolyte disturbances, especially hypokalaemia, hypomagnesaemia and hypercalcaemia.

A4   A

Adrenaline (epinephrine) is a sympathomimetic agent that causes bronchodilatation. It is used to relieve bronchospasm in anaphylactic shock reactions. Histamine, kinins and prostaglandins, such as prostaglandin E_2, are inflammatory mediators. In response to allergic stimuli, inflammatory mediators may cause bronchoconstrictions. Guaifenesin is an expectorant preparation that increases bronchial secretions to promote the expulsion of the mucus coughed up.

A5   B

Information sources recommended to be available in a pharmacy include a recent copy of a drug formulary, such as the *British National Formulary;* a current edition of a drug compendium, such as *Martindale: The Complete Drug Reference;* a copy of a pharmacology and therapeutics reference, such as Goodman and Gilman's *Pharmacological Basis of Therapeutics* and an updated copy of the laws regulating the pharmacy profession.

A6   A

Clarinase contains the non-sedating antihistamine loratadine and the nasal decongestant pseudoephedrine. Similarly to Clarinase, Cirrus contains a non-sedating antihistamine cetirizine and the nasal decongestant pseudoephedrine. Actifed contains the sedating antihistamine triprolidine and the nasal decongestant pseudoephedrine. Clarityn, Xyzal and Telfast contain a non-sedating antihistamine, namely loratadine, levocetirizine and fexofenadine respectively.

A7   C

Threadworm infections are caused by *Enterobius vermicularis*. The infestation starts when the patient ingests the worm's ova, which then hatch and infect the small intestine. The female threadworms migrate to the caecum and anus so that at night they lay their eggs in the perianal area. The eggs produce a sticky secretion and attach themselves to the skin. It is the sticky secretion that causes the itchiness that is the main symptom. Enterobiasis, as the condition is known, is treated with the administration of anthelmintics. A single dose is administered. However, as re-infestation is common, a second dose given after 2–3 weeks is recommended. A warm bath taken first thing in the morning is often recommended to remove ova laid during the night.

A8   B

Cold remedies aim to relieve cold symptoms and very often contain a combination of an analgesic, a sedating antihistamine, a nasal decongestant and ascorbic acid. Beecham's Hot Lemon and Honey sachets are a cold remedy preparation containing paracetamol, ascorbic acid and the nasal decongestant phenylephrine. Otrivine drops are a topical preparation containing the nasal decongestant xylometazoline. It is indicated for nasal congestion. Atarax tablets contain the sedating antihistamine hydroxyzine, which is used in pruritus and for the short-term management of anxiety. Actifed Compound Linctus is a cough preparation containing the sedating antihistamine triprolidine, the nasal decongestant pseudoephedrine and the cough suppressant dextromethorpan. It is therefore indicated in dry cough. Karvol inhalation capsules contain levomenthol with chlorbutanol, pine oils, terpineol and thymol and are meant to relieve sinusitis.

A9   B

Acetazolamide is a carbonic anhydrase inhibitor that reduces aqueous humour production and is therefore indicated in glaucoma to reduce the intraocular pressure. Salbutamol is a selective, short-acting $beta_2$-agonist used as a bronchodilator in asthma. Tolbutamide is a short-acting sulphonylurea used in type 2 (non-insulin dependent) diabetes mellitus. Chlorpromazine is an aliphatic neuroleptic antipsychotic drug used in schizophrenia. Zafirlukast is a leukotriene-receptor antagonist that is indicated in the prophylaxis of asthma but should not be used to relieve acute severe asthma.

A10   C

Isordil is a proprietary (trade name) preparation of isosorbide dinitrate, a nitrate. Sildenafil, the active ingredient of Viagra, interacts with nitrates and the two active ingredients should not be administered concurrently, as a significant hypotensive effect may occur.

A11   A

Famciclovir is the prodrug of penciclovir and is indicated in the treatment of chickenpox and genital herpes.

A12   B

Ergotamine is an ergot alkaloid indicated in the treatment of migraine. Ergotamine has marked vasoconstrictor effects.

A13   E

Hydrocortisone for intravenous administration is available as the sodium succinate salt.

A14   D

Lasilix containing furosemide is classified as a loop diuretic and acts by inhibiting re-absorption from the ascending part of the loop of Henle. Thiazide diuretics, such as bendroflumethiazide, act by inhibiting re-absorption at the beginning of the distal convoluted tubule.

A15   B

Unlike seborrhoeic dermatitis, chloasma, acne vulgaris and herpes simplex labialis, furuncles (boils) are not worsened by skin exposure.

A16   E

Flagyl (metronidazole, antimicrobial agent) tablets are available in 200 mg and 400 mg strengths. Istin (amlodipine, a dihydropyridine calcium-channel blocker) is available as 5 mg and 10 mg tablets. Risperdal (risperidone, atypical antipsychotic) is available as tablets of 500 µg, 1 mg, 2 mg, 3 mg, 4 mg and 6 mg strengths. Naprosyn (naproxen, a non-steroidal anti-inflammatory drug) is available as Naprosyn 250 mg and 500 mg capsules. Migril, the antimigraine tablets contain ergotamine 2 mg (ergot alkaloid), cyclizine 50 mg (antihistamine with anti-emetic properties) and caffeine 100 mg (weak stimulant).

A17   C

Triamcinolone is a corticosteroid that is more potent than hydrocortisone and has a longer duration of action. Triamcinolone has only slight mineralocorticoid activity, whereas hydrocortisone has high mineralocorticoid activity and therefore triamcinolone is unsuitable for disease suppression on a long-term basis. Triamcinolone is available as injection, dental paste, nasal spray and as cream or ointment preparations. Hydrocortisone is available as cream, tablets and injections.

A18   D

Vaginal infections caused by fungi (vaginal candidiasis) are best treated with topical preparations containing imidazoles. Generally, pessaries are preferred to cream formulations. Gyno-Daktarin pessary contains miconazole (imidazole antifungal). Canesten cream containing clotrimazole (imidazole antifungal) would be an alternative to the pessary. In case of recurrence, a single dose of oral fluconazole (triazole antifungal) 150 mg capsule may be effective. Betadine douche containing povidone-iodine is less effective than the imidazole preparations. Ortho-Gynest cream contains estriol, which is used in vaginal atrophy in post-menopausal women. Lamisil tablets containing terbinafine are not indicated in vaginal candidiasis.

A19   D

Omeprazole and rabeprazole inhibit gastric acid formation by blocking the hydrogen–potassium ATPase pump hence the name proton pump inhibitors. Misoprostol is a synthetic prostaglandin analogue having antisecretory properties, thus helping in the healing of gastric ulcers. Misoprostol is used in elderly patients taking non-steroidal anti-inflammatory drugs and in patients in whom the non-steroidal anti-inflammatory drugs cannot be discontinued. Ranitidine decreases the gastric acid output by antagonising the histamine H_2-receptor. Proton pump inhibitors, misoprostol and H_2-receptor antagonists can all be used in the treatment and prophylaxis of gastric ulcers. Loperamide is an antidiarrhoeal agent.

A20 A

Cradle cap is a form of seborrhoeic dermatitis of the scalp presenting in babies up to 3 months of age. The condition appears as scales and crusts on the baby's scalp. It is not contagious and, although it tends to affect babies with a predisposition to food allergy, cradle cap is not a food allergy. The condition, which may be associated with nappy rash, resolves spontaneously within a year. First-line treatment is the application of almond oil, arachis oil or baby oil on to the scalp, leaving it overnight and then washing it off the next day.

A21 A

The structure is an 18-carbon steroid and represents estradiol, an oestrogen.

A22 E

Daktarin cream containing the imidazole antifungal miconazole, is a brand marketed by Janssen-Cilag.

A23 B

Otrivine drops containing the nasal decongestant xylometazoline, is a brand marketed by Novartis.

A24 D

Rhinocort Aqua is the proprietary preparation of a topical nasal spray containing the corticosteroid budesonide and is marketed by AstraZeneca.

A25   A

Buscopan contains hyoscine butylbromide, which is a quaternary ammonium compound with antimuscarinic properties. It is used as an antispasmodic and therefore may be useful in irritable bowel syndrome. Hyoscine butylbromide, as with all antimuscarinics, must be used with caution in patients with prostatic hypertrophy, as they may lead to urinary retention.

A26   C

Voltarol is a proprietary preparation of diclofenac. Diclofenac, like all the non-steroidal anti-inflammatory drugs, may lead to bronchoconstriction (particularly when used systemically) and therefore must be used with caution in asthma.

A27   D

Natrilix is a proprietary preparation of indapamide, a thiazide diuretic and hence may cause gout as a side-effect.

A28   A

Acetazolamide is a carbonic anhydrase inhibitor, used primarily in glaucoma to reduce aqueous humour production. Acetazolamide may cause blood disorders including agranulocytosis (deficiency of neutrophils) as a side-effect.

A29   B

Amoxicillin is a broad spectrum penicillin antibiotic. Antibiotics tend to cause pseudomembranous colitis as a result of colonisation of the colon by *Clostridium difficile* following antibiotic therapy.

A30   C

Atracurium is a non-depolarising muscle relaxant, which may cause respiratory depression as a side-effect.

A31 A

Doxorubicin is a chemotherapeutic anthracycline antibiotic, which may cause cardiotoxicity through the free-radical mechanism. Cardiotoxicity limits the clinical usefulness as a result of which doxorubicin has a total cumulative dose of about 450 mg/m^2 body surface area. Patients with pre-existing cardiac disease, elderly patients and patients who have received myocardial irradiation must be treated cautiously and cardiac monitoring may be required.

A32 B

Methotrexate is an antimetabolite chemotherapeutic agent, which may also be used for severe resistant psoriasis. The dose is usually administered orally once a week. Haematological and biochemical parameters are monitored throughout treatment.

A33 D

Cyclophosphamide is an antineoplastic agent that causes DNA cross-linking and abnormal base-pairing through a mechanism called alkylation, hence the name alkylating agent. Cyclophosphamide may also be used in resistant rheumatoid arthritis.

A34 E

Optrex preparations contain witch hazel, which has both astringent and anti-inflammatory properties. It is indicated for sore and tired eyes.

A35 A

Suboxone contains buprenorphine, an opioid partial agonist used in opioid dependence in combination with naloxone.

A36 B

Anadin Extra contains paracetamol, aspirin and caffeine, the latter being a mild stimulant that increases the absorption and activity of the analgesics, paracetamol and aspirin.

A37 A

Sumatriptan is a $5HT_1$ agonist, which is indicated in the treatment of acute migraine attacks. Sumatriptan may cause vasoconstriction as a side-effect and therefore its use is reserved for patients in whom other conventional migraine analgesics have failed.

A38 C

Tramadol is an opioid analgesic, which acts by exerting an opioid effect and through the stimulation of adrenergic and serotonin pathways. Compared with the other opioids, tramadol is less likely to cause the typical opioid side-effects, such as respiratory depression, and constipation. It is also less likely to cause addiction.

A39 A

Sumatriptan, a $5HT_1$ agonist, is contraindicated in ischaemic heart disease as it may cause vasoconstriction, leading to chest tightness, and precipitating ischaemic heart disease.

A40 B

Ondansetron is a $5HT_3$ antagonist, blocking serotonin receptors in the central nervous system and the gastrointestinal tract. It is useful in the management of postoperative nausea and vomiting associated with cytotoxics.

A41 A

The antiviral aciclovir cream is available as 5%. It is indicated in the treatment of herpes simplex infections.

A42 B

Mupirocin is a broad spectrum antibiotic available as a 2% ointment.

A43   C

Azelaic acid, which has antimicrobial and anticomedonal properties, is available as 20% cream indicated for use in acne.

A44   D

Fluticasone cream is a corticosteroid preparation available as 0.05%.

A45   C

Mobic is the proprietary preparation of meloxicam, a non-steroidal anti-inflammatory drug, which is also a selective inhibitor of cyclo-oxygenase-2. It is therefore less likely to cause gastrointestinal side-effects than other non-steroidal anti-inflammatory drugs. However, it is still best to administer meloxicam after food.

A46   B

Vermox is the proprietary preparation of mebendazole, which is an anthelmintic. A single dose of mebendazole is indicated in the management of threadworms, with a second dose 2–3 weeks later avoiding re-infection, which tends to be common.

A47   A

Colofac is the proprietary preparation of mebeverine, which is an antispasmodic useful in irritable bowel syndrome. Mebeverine is a direct relaxant of the smooth muscle and, unlike hyoscine, is not an antimuscarinic.

A48   E

Circadin is the proprietary preparation of melatonin, which is used for the short-term management of insomnia.

A49   B

Alfuzosin is a selective alpha$_1$–blocker, which relaxes the smooth muscle in benign prostatic hyperplasia and hence increases the urinary outflow.

Alpha-blockers tend to cause vasodilation leading to hypotension especially after the first dose. Subsequently patients on alpha-blockers are advised to take the first dose at night before retiring to bed. Alpha-blockers also tend to cause drowsiness so patients are advised to be careful when driving.

A50   B

Venlafaxine is a serotonin and noradrenaline re-uptake inhibitor indicated in depression and may be used in generalised anxiety disorder. Venlafaxine can cause diarrhoea and headache as side-effects. It does not cause blurred vision.

A51   A

The dose of aciclovir in patients with renal impairment should be reduced as aciclovir is eliminated by the renal system. Most penicillins are eliminated by the renal system and hence dose reduction of amoxicillin is required in cases of renal impairment. Non-steroidal anti-inflammatory drugs cause the inhibition of the biosynthesis of prostaglandins involved in the maintenance of renal blood flow. This may precipitate acute renal insufficiency in patients with renal impairment. Furthermore non-steroidal anti-inflammatory drugs tend to cause water and sodium retention and hence aggrevate renal impairment.

A52   B

Phenytoin is an anti-epileptic drug. Patients taking anti-epileptic drugs are advised to take the medicine routinely, as directed, to stabilise and to avoid epileptic attacks as much as possible. Phenytoin has a narrow therapeutic index so it is important to identify side-effects. It may cause blood disorders. Patients are therefore advised to report immediately any symptoms of bruising or unexplained bleeding. Visual symptoms as a result of phenytoin do not commonly occur. Their occurrence may indicate overdosage.

A53   D

Endometriosis refers to the abnormal presence of endometrial tissue growing outside the uterus in places such as the abdomen, the peritoneum, ovary and the bladder. Symptoms of endometriosis include infertility. Pelvic pain may occur before or during menses.

A54 B

The polio vaccine is administered in three doses at 1-month intervals, starting from the age of 2 months. The pertussis vaccine is given in combination with the diphtheria and tetanus vaccines as a 3-in-1 vaccine, the DTP vaccine. The DTP vaccine follows the schedule of the polio vaccine, so at 2 months, the DTP and the polio vaccine are given. Both are repeated at 3 months of age and at 4 months of age. In areas where the incidence of tuberculosis is not greater than 40 per 100 000, the BCG vaccine is not usually recommended for infants of 0–6 months.

A55 E

Gastro-oesophageal reflux in infants is common and tends to resolve at 12–18 months of age. Simple procedures, such as posture and thickening of foods, may help to alleviate gastro-oesophageal disease in infants.

A56 A

Clinical signs of dehydration in children include tachycardia, loss of skin turgor and dry tongue.

A57 B

Mumps is an acute viral infection transmitted by airborne droplets. Mumps is considered to be a childhood infection affecting those between 5 and 15 years of age. Classic symptoms of mumps include fever, chills, malaise, and enlargement of the parotid glands, which may be unilateral or bilateral. The swelling of the parotid glands may result in the patient experiencing a dry mouth because saliva flow is blocked.

A58   C

Characteristic symptoms of allergic rhinitis (hay fever) include itchy nose, prolonged sneezing attacks, rhinorrhoea and red, itchy eyes (conjunctival lacrimation).

A59   E

Cataracts refer to the opacity of the lens of the eye or of its capsule. Symptoms of cataracts are a progressive decrease in visual acuity as the lens becomes visibly opaque. Cataracts are usually painless but pain may be an accompanying symptom if the cataract swells and secondary glaucoma develops.

A60   C

Calcipotriol is a vitamin D derivative used topically for psoriasis. It does not cause skin discoloration and does not stain clothes.

A61   B

Ciclosporin is a potent immunosuppressant, which is markedly nephrotoxic. It may cause gastrointestinal disturbances. Ciclosporin is available as capsules, oral solution and parenteral preparations.

A62   A

As with other quinolones, ciprofloxacin should be used with caution in epileptic patients (since it may precipitate seizures), in children, during pregnancy and breast-feeding (due to risk of arthropathy in weight-bearing joints).

A63   A

Arthrotec tablets contain the non-steroidal anti-inflammatory drug diclofenac and the prostaglandin misoprostol. The combination of the two active ingredients makes Arthrotec suitable in patients predisposed to gastrointestinal ulceration. Dulco-lax (bisacodyl) tablets act as a stimulant laxative. Voltarol Retard tablets contain the non-steroidal anti-inflammatory drug diclofenac. All three preparations must be swallowed whole without being chewed, either because of the nature of the active ingredient (misoprostol, bisacodyl) or because the product is a modified-release preparation (Voltarol Retard tablets).

A64   E

Ranitidine is a H_2-receptor antagonist, which reduces the gastric output. Unlike cimetidine, ranitidine does not interact with cytochrome P450, so does not retard hepatic metabolism of certain drugs, such as warfarin. Ranitidine may be administered as 150 mg twice daily or 300 mg at night.

A65   C

Both omeprazole, a proton pump inhibitor and paclitaxel, a taxane cytotoxic may cause nausea and vomiting as side-effects. Prednisolone, as with other corticosteroids, does not cause nausea and vomiting. Corticosteroids such as dexamethasone are administered to relieve nausea and vomiting, particularly that associated with chemotherapy.

A66   A

Levodopa is the amino precursor of dopamine. It is used to replenish depleted dopamine in Parkinson's disease. Levodopa may cause insomnia, reddish discoloration of urine and headache.

A67   A

Heparins can be used during pregnancy for the management of thrombo-embolic disease because they do not cross the placenta. Administration of heparins should be stopped at onset of labour. Low molecular weight heparins are preferred during pregnancy since they pose lower risks of osteoporosis and of heparin-induced thrombocytopenia.

A68   B

Headaches that are constantly painful and seem to be particularly worse in the morning may be associated with uncontrolled hypertension. Patients presenting with headaches accompanied by fever and neck stiffness should be referred.

A69 C

Periodontitis is a dental condition caused by bacteria where plaque-induced inflammatory changes affect the periodontal ligament and the alveolar bone leading to loss of the periodontal structure and resorption of the alveolar bone. Periodontitis that, unlike gingivitis, is not reversible, tends to be chronic and requires referral.

A70 C

Cystitis is a urinary tract bacterial infection generally caused by *Escherichia coli*. It results in inflammation of the bladder and urethra and is characterised by a frequent urge to pass urine accompanied by a burning or stinging sensation on urination. Cystitis is common in females but less common in men who must always be referred. Children are always referred as urinary tract infections make children susceptible to permanent kidney and bladder damage. Management of cystitis is based on the administration of alkalinising agents to help restore the pH of the urine to normal non-acidic environment. The alkalinising agents are administered three times daily for two days and the risk of hyperkalaemia is negligible.

A71 C

Tamoxifen is an oestrogen-receptor antagonist indicated as adjuvant hormonal treatment in oestrogen-receptor-positive breast cancer in postmenopausal women. Common side-effects include alopecia and uterine fibroids.

A72 E

In nicotine replacement therapy, the chewing gum releases nicotine, which is absorbed through the buccal mucosa every time a piece of chewing gum is chewed. The chewing gum is chewed for 30 minutes, only when one feels the urge to smoke. The transdermal patch provides a residual nicotine level throughout the application. A side-effect of nicotine chewing gum may be aphthous ulcers.

A73 E

Zolpidem is an imidazopyridine but not a benzodiazepine; however, it acts on the same receptors as benzodiazepines. Zolpidem has a short duration of action and is indicated for patients who have difficulty sleeping. It does not have any hangover effects. The dose of Zolpidem should be reduced in patients with hepatic impairment and it should be avoided in cases of severe hepatic impairment.

A74 E

Orciprenaline is a partially selective adrenoceptor-agonist and hence it is more likely to have effects on the cardiovascular system, such as arrhythmias, than the selective adrenoceptor-agonists, such as salbutamol, terbutaline and the long-acting beta-agonists salmeterol and formoterol. Orciprenaline is available only as tablets or syrup and can be prescribed to 4-year-old children.

A75 C

Gliclazide is a sulphonylurea. Gliclazide has a short half-life, unlike glibenclamide. For this reason elderly patients are often given gliclazide, to avoid hypoglycaemic attacks, which are more often associated with long-acting sulphonylureas. Fluconazole (triazole antifungal) interacts with the sulphonylureas by increasing the plasma concentration of sulphonylureas when both drugs are administered concomitantly.

A76 E

Typhoid fever is caused by *Salmonella typhii* bacilli. The condition has an incubation period of about 5–23 days. Classic symptoms of typhoid fever include headache, abdominal pain with constipation or diarrhoea. Rose-coloured spots and macular rashes on the abdomen are characteristic of typhoid fever.

A77 B

Largactil is a proprietary preparation of chlorpromazine, an aliphatic antipsychotic with marked sedation and moderate antimuscarinic and extrapyramidal side-effects. Serenace is a proprietary preparation of haloperidol, a butyrophenone antipsychotic with marked extrapyramidal side-effects, moderate sedation but not very likely to cause hypotension. Tegretol is a proprietary preparation of carbamazepine, an anti-epileptic drug indicated in partial and secondary generalised tonic-clonic seizures, primary generalised tonic-clonic seizures, trigeminal neuralgia and in the prophylaxis of bipolar disorder unresponsive to lithium.

A78 D

Prophylaxis for malaria includes the administration of antimalarial tablets and protection against mosquito bites but does not include any vaccinations. Hepatitis C is a viral infection and no vaccine is available. Hepatitis B is a viral infection and prophylaxis is provided by a vaccine.

A79 B

Griseofulvin and terbinafine are indicated in the management of fungal nail infections. Nystatin (polyene antifungal) is indicated in the management of *Candida* infections and is not indicated for fungal nail infections.

A80 A

According to Cardiovascular Risk Prediction Charts (BNF 2009), an elderly, non-diabetic, male smoker has a cardiovascular risk of 10–20% over the next 10 years. The use of statins to control hyperlipidaemia and reduce risk is recommended.

A81 C

Ephedrine is a vasoconstrictor sympathomimetic agent that causes an increase in blood pressure and an increase in heart rate. It is used in spinal or epidural anaesthesia where it is administered by slow intravenous injection to reverse the resultant hypotension caused by the sympathetic block induced by the anaesthesia.

A82   B

Buccastem is a proprietary preparation of prochlorperazine buccal tablets. Patient is advised to leave the tablet to dissolve after it is placed high between upper lip and gum. Prochlorperazine is a phenothiazine that acts as an anti-emetic by blocking the chemoreceptor trigger zone in the brain. It is used for the prophylaxis and management of nausea and vomiting associated with emetogenic drugs (cytotoxic chemotherapy, opioids, anaesthesia), migraine and vestibular disorders. The buccal tablet results in absorption of the drug through the buccal mucosa, thus bypassing the stomach.

A83   D

Flumazenil is a benzodiazepine antagonist that is used in anaesthesia for the reversal of central sedative effects of benzodiazepines. It should not be administered rapidly so as to avoid patient wakening too rapidly, which can lead to agitation, anxiety, fear and convulsions, particularly in high-risk patients, e.g. those with a history of epilepsy or head injury.

A84   C

Orlistat is a pancreatic lipase inhibitor used in conjunction with a hypocaloric diet to reduce the absorption of dietary fat in obese patients. Orlistat is administered twice daily immediately before, during or up to 1 hour after each meal. If the meal contains no fat there is no need to take Orlistat.

A85   A

All angiotensin-converting enzyme inhibitors including enalapril, may precipitate a hypoglycaemic attack in a diabetic patient because they may potentiate the effect of sulphonylureas.

A86   E

Repaglinide is a newer oral hypoglycaemic agent, indicated in type 2 diabetes either in combination with metformin or as monotherapy. Repaglinide stimulates insulin release.

A87   E

Urinalysis for glucose monitoring can detect hyperglycaemia but not hypoglycaemia. Blood glucose monitoring gives a direct measure of the glucose concentration at the time of the test. It can detect both hyperglycaemia and hypoglycaemia and it is used in preference to urinalysis. Random blood glucose concentrations must be maintained at 7.8 mmol/L (140 mg/dL) but the level is expected to rise post-prandially.

A88   D

Both budesonide and fluticasone are corticosteroids but fluticasone is more potent than budesonide and has a higher first-pass effect, hence more of the drug is metabolised leading to fewer adverse effects. A dose of 100 µg of budesonide is equivalent to 50 µg of fluticasone. Both budesonide and fluticasone are indicated for the prophylaxis of allergic rhinitis (hay fever).

A89   B

Xalatan drops is a proprietary preparation of latanoprost (prostaglandin analogue), indicated in glaucoma.

A90   A

Xalatan (latanoprost) is a prostaglandin analogue, which increases the uvoscleral outflow, thereby decreasing the intraocular pressure. The drops, which are applied once daily, preferably in the evening, may cause eye discoloration especially in patients with mixed colour irides.

A91–94

Imipramine is a tricyclic antidepressant (TCA), which acts by blocking the re-uptake of serotonin and noradrenaline. TCAs may cause cardiovascular side-effects including arrhythmias and heart block. There is no interaction between imipramine and angiotensin-converting enzyme inhibitors such as perindopril, which can be used as a first-line treatment in the management of hypertension. The risk of postural hypotension occurring as a result of the use of diuretics such as bendroflumethiazide (thiazide diuretic) is increased in patients who are taking imipramine. Plasma concentration of imipramine is increased with concomitant administration of propranolol (beta-blocker). Furosemide is a loop diuretic that is not normally recommended in the management of hypertension.

A91 2

A92 4

A93 1

A94 3

A95 B

Zestril contains lisinopril, an angiotensin-converting enzyme inhibitor. Angiotensin-converting enzyme inhibitors tend to retain potassium, thereby counteracting the potassium loss caused by the thiazide diuretic bendroflumethiazide.

A96 C

Concomitant administration of methotrexate and Voltarol, a proprietary preparation of diclofenac, a non-steroidal anti-inflammatory drug, may result in accumulation of methotrexate as its excretion is reduced. The use of diclofenac and diuretics such as bendroflumethiazide may increase the risk of nephrotoxicity. Concomitant use of alcohol and an angiotensin-converting enzyme inhibitor such as lisinopril (Zestril) may result in an enhanced hypotensive effect. Alcohol and the benzodiazepine diazepam (Valium) may result in enhanced sedation.

A97   B

Methotrexate is a cytotoxic agent that may cause pulmonary toxicity and therefore patients are advised to contact the doctor if cough develops.

Also occurrence of cough may indicate a bacterial respiratory tract infection that requires antibacterial therapy. Patients who are receiving methotrexate may experience a drop in white-cell count, making them more susceptible to infections.

A98   A

Methotrexate is an antimetabolite, which is metabolised by the renal and hepatic systems and may lead to renal and hepatic toxicities. Liver and renal function tests are therefore carried out for patients who are administered the drug. Methotrexate can lead to myelosuppression and therefore full blood counts must be monitored for patients taking it.

A99   D

Methotrexate is one of the disease-modifying antirheumatic drugs, which are administered once a week. The initial dose is 7.5 mg administered once a week and the maximum dose is 15–20 mg administered once a week.

A100 A

Deltacortil is a proprietary preparation of the corticosteroid prednisolone. As with other corticosteroids, prednisolone may lead to precipitation of osteoporosis, insomnia and candidiasis.

Test 3

Questions

Questions 1–18

Directions: Each of the questions or incomplete statements is followed by five suggested answers. Select the best answer in each case.

Q1 The refrigerator in the pharmacy that is used for storage of pharmaceutical products should be kept at a temperature of:

A ❑ 0–3°C
B ❑ 2–8°C
C ❑ 5–10°C
D ❑ 6–12°C
E ❑ −3–8°C

Q2 A patient with diverticular disease is instructed to take a laxative. The pharmacist should appropriately recommend:

A ❑ Senokot tablets
B ❑ Dulco-lax tablets
C ❑ glycerol suppositories
D ❑ Fybogel sachets
E ❑ magnesium hydroxide mixture

Q3 A patient comes into the pharmacy with rhinorrhoea. Which of the following list of symptoms is most likely to indicate allergic rhinitis?

A ❑ coloured sputum
B ❑ fever
C ❑ sore throat
D ❑ sneezing
E ❑ malaise

Q4   What is the dose of mefenamic acid that can be given to a child of 3 years with a body weight of 15 kg, considering that the dosing regimen is 25 mg/kg daily in divided doses?

A   ❑ 10 mL t.d.s.
B   ❑ 5 mL t.d.s.
C   ❑ 2.5 mL t.d.s.
D   ❑ 5 mL b.d.
E   ❑ 7 mL t.d.s.

Q5   Which of the following products could be responsible for causing constipation?

A   ❑ Naprosyn
B   ❑ Adalat
C   ❑ co-codamol
D   ❑ Amoxil
E   ❑ Dulco-lax

Q6   Over-the-counter products that may be recommended to prevent napkin dermatitis include all EXCEPT:

A   ❑ zinc and castor oil ointment
B   ❑ Vasogen
C   ❑ Sudocrem
D   ❑ Canesten HC
E   ❑ Drapolene

Q7   A physician calls the pharmacist and enquires about a sustained-release NSAID for a patient who has sciatica. Of the following products, the pharmacist could suggest:

A   ❑ Nu-seals tablets
B   ❑ fentanyl patches
C   ❑ co-codamol tablets
D   ❑ Voltarol tablets
E   ❑ Suboxone tablets

Q8   When comparing amlodipine and nifedipine, amlodipine:

A   ❏ has a longer duration of action
B   ❏ can be used in hypertension
C   ❏ is available as a spray formulation
D   ❏ causes ankle swelling as a side-effect
E   ❏ cannot be used in angina

Q9   A microorganism that is associated with serious complications if associated with eye infections is:

A   ❏ herpes simplex virus
B   ❏ *Escherichia coli*
C   ❏ *Pseudomonas aeruginosa*
D   ❏ *Aspergillus niger*
E   ❏ *Bacillus subtilis*

Q10   Gingivitis refers to inflammation of the:

A   ❏ pharynx
B   ❏ tongue
C   ❏ gums
D   ❏ larynx
E   ❏ salivary gland

Q11   Which of the following is NOT an inflammatory mediator?

A   ❏ bradykinin
B   ❏ histamine
C   ❏ lymphokines
D   ❏ glucose
E   ❏ lysosomal enzymes

Q12   Otitis media is caused by the following microorganisms EXCEPT:

A   ❑ *Staphylococcus aureus*
B   ❑ *Haemophilus influenzae*
C   ❑ *Streptococcus pyogenes*
D   ❑ *Pseudomonas aeruginosa*
E   ❑ *Enterobius vermicularis*

Q13   Which of the following drugs is associated with precipitation of a migraine attack?

A   ❑ aspirin
B   ❑ combined oral contraceptives
C   ❑ metoclopramide
D   ❑ propranolol
E   ❑ diazepam

Q14   Which of the following is NOT a cytotoxic drug?

A   ❑ vincristine
B   ❑ fluorouracil
C   ❑ ciclosporin
D   ❑ bleomycin
E   ❑ methotrexate

Q15   Legionnaire's disease affects primarily the:

A   ❑ respiratory system
B   ❑ urinary tract
C   ❑ skin
D   ❑ eye
E   ❑ gums

Q16   Gingival hyperplasia is associated with:

A   ❏ digoxin
B   ❏ phenytoin
C   ❏ enalapril
D   ❏ theophylline
E   ❏ captopril

Q17   A patient comes to the pharmacy with mosquito bites. Which of the following preparations would be most suitable?

A   ❏ paracetamol tablets
B   ❏ hydrocortisone cream
C   ❏ fusidic acid cream
D   ❏ benzocaine spray
E   ❏ mepyramine cream

Q18   The molecular structure of ampicillin is shown below.

This structure may be modified to produce amoxicillin by attaching a (an):

A   ❏ hydroxyl group
B   ❏ amide
C   ❏ aldehyde
D   ❏ hydroxyl group and carboxylic group
E   ❏ hydroxyl group and chloride group

Questions 19–31

Directions: Each group of questions below consists of five lettered headings followed by a list of numbered questions. For each numbered question select the one heading that is most closely related to it. Each heading may be used once, more than once, or not at all.

Questions 19–23 concern the use of the following drugs in patients with renal impairment:

A   ❏ clarithromycin
B   ❏ clindamycin
C   ❏ co-amoxiclav
D   ❏ fusidic acid
E   ❏ gentamicin

Select, from A to E, which one of the above:

Q19   should be avoided in modified-release oral preparation if creatinine clearance is less than 30 mL/minute

Q20   has a risk of crystalluria with high doses, particularly during parenteral therapy

Q21   requires earlier and more frequent measurement of drug serum concentrations than in patients with normal renal function

Q22   requires no caution in patients with renal impairment

Q23   is excreted principally via the kidney and accumulation occurs in renal impairment

Questions 24–26 concern the following drugs:

A ❑ metoclopramide
B ❑ promethazine
C ❑ cinnarizine
D ❑ cyclizine
E ❑ hyoscine

Select, from A to E, which one of the above:

Q24 is ineffective in motion sickness

Q25 can be recommended for motion sickness when a sedative effect is desired

Q26 acts on the chemoreceptor trigger zone

Questions 27–31 concern the following cautionary labels:

A ❑ 'May cause drowsiness. If affected do not drive or operate machinery'
B ❑ 'Swallowed whole, not chewed'
C ❑ 'Avoid exposure of skin to direct sunlight or sunlamps'
D ❑ 'Avoid alcoholic drink'
E ❑ 'Take an hour before food or on an empty stomach'

Select, from A to E, which one of the above should be used when dispensing:

Q27 Dulco-lax tablets

Q28 Slow-K tablets

Q29 Zaditen syrup

Q30 Flagyl tablets

Q31 flucloxacillin capsules

Questions 32–80

Directions: For each of the questions below, ONE or MORE of the responses is (are) correct. Decide which of the responses is (are) correct. Then choose:

A   ❏ if 1, 2 and 3 are correct
B   ❏ if 1 and 2 only are correct
C   ❏ if 2 and 3 only are correct
D   ❏ if 1 only is correct
E   ❏ if 3 only is correct

Directions summarised				
A	**B**	**C**	**D**	**E**
1, 2, 3	1, 2 only	2, 3 only	1 only	3 only

Q32   Thrombocytopenia:

1   ❏ may arise after 5–10 days of administration of heparin
2   ❏ results in spontaneous haemorrhage
3   ❏ requires intravenous administration of factor VIII

Q33   Patients receiving atomoxetine therapy should be advised:

1   ❏ that tics may occur as a common side-effect
2   ❏ to report agitation or irritability
3   ❏ to seek prompt medical attention if abdominal pain, darkening of urine or unexplained nausea occur

Q34   Aripiprazole:

1   ❏ may cause impotence
2   ❏ causes little or no elevation of prolactin
3   ❏ may precipitate suicidal ideation

Q35   Trastuzumab:

1   ❑ is effective in breast cancer that overexpresses human epidermal growth factor receptor-2 (HER2)
2   ❑ may be associated with the occurrence of chills, fever and hypersensitivity reactions as a result of intravenous infusion of the drug
3   ❑ is always administered in combination with doxorubicin

Q36   Suboxone:

1   ❑ contains naloxone, which is a specific opioid antagonist
2   ❑ is available as sublingual tablets
3   ❑ may cause drowsiness

Q37   Care should be taken with the use of the following drugs in a patient with hepatic impairment:

1   ❑ statins
2   ❑ antihistamines
3   ❑ selective serotonin re-uptake inhibitors

Q38   Drugs that can significantly interact adversely with calcium-channel blockers include:

1   ❑ atenolol
2   ❑ ranitidine
3   ❑ gliclazide

Q39   Products that should be stored in a refrigerator include:

1   ❑ Varilrix
2   ❑ Daktacort cream
3   ❑ Sofradex eye drops

Q40   A patient with hypertension (male 56 years, weight 55 kg) visits the pharmacy with a new prescription for diclofenac. The patient is already taking enalapril 20 mg daily, atenolol 100 mg daily and

bendroflumethiazide   2.5 mg   daily.   Which   of   the   following
statement(s) is (are) true?

1   ❑ the patient may experience a hypotensive reaction
2   ❑ the patient may experience a hypertensive reaction
3   ❑ there is an increased risk of nephrotoxicity

Q41   Ivabradine

1   ❑ causes tachycardia
2   ❑ is indicated in patients with an acute myocardial infarction
3   ❑ may lead to blurred vision

Q42   When testing body fluids in a pharmacy, it is recommended that:

1   ❑ tests are carried out in a designated area in the pharmacy
2   ❑ contaminated waste is disposed of in an appropriate dustbin
3   ❑ test is undertaken after opening hours

Q43   Which of the following statement(s) is (are) correct about omeprazole?

1   ❑ it   inhibits   gastric   acid   by   blocking   the   hydrogen–
potassium adenosine triphosphate enzyme system of the gastric parietal cell
2   ❑ side-effects expected include diarrhoea, headache, nausea
and vomiting
3   ❑ concomitant use with phenytoin is associated with enhanced
effects of phenytoin

Q44   Which of the following statement(s) is (are) true about digoxin?

1   ❑ it has a long half-life
2   ❑ side-effects include nausea, vomiting, diarrhoea, abdominal
pain, arrhythmias
3   ❑ a   geriatric   dosage   formulation   is   available   as   62.5 µg
tablets

Q45   Patients taking amiodarone should be advised to:

1   ❑ avoid exposure to sunlight
2   ❑ use a sun protection lotion daily
3   ❑ be careful when driving at night

Q46   When dispensing simvastatin, the patient should be advised to:

1   ❑ report promptly unexplained muscle pain, tenderness and weakness
2   ❑ take dose at night
3   ❑ follow dietary measures

Q47   Sumatriptan should be used with caution in patients:

1   ❑ with a history of angina
2   ❑ taking fluoxetine
3   ❑ taking enalapril maleate

Q48   Doxycycline:

1   ❑ is contraindicated in children under 12 years
2   ❑ cannot be used in patients with kidney disease
3   ❑ is only active against Gram-positive organisms

Q49   Which of the following drugs should be avoided in breast-feeding?

1   ❑ aspirin
2   ❑ diazepam
3   ❑ amoxicillin

Q50   Referral is warranted when a patient presents with a headache that is:

1   ❑ accompanied by nausea, vomiting and nose bleeds
2   ❑ accompanied by paraesthesia, numbness
3   ❑ unilateral

Q51   Croup:

1   ❑ occurs in young children
2   ❑ is characterised by a barking cough
3   ❑ may lead to cyanosis and respiratory failure

Q52   Verrucas:

1   ❑ are caused by the human papilloma virus
2   ❑ are characterised by a cauliflower-like appearance
3   ❑ may be contracted in swimming pools and public baths

Q53   Hiatus hernia:

1   ❑ is the protrusion of a portion of the stomach into the thorax
2   ❑ may be asymptomatic
3   ❑ is common in obese patients

Q54   Gluten-free products are recommended to patients with:

1   ❑ coeliac disease
2   ❑ diabetes mellitus
3   ❑ liver disease

Q55   Chilblains:

1   ❑ are local inflammatory lesions
2   ❑ occur in cold conditions
3   ❑ are accompanied by intense pruritus

Q56   Migraine headache:

1   ❑ may be precipitated by ingestion of chocolate
2   ❑ may be preceded by an aura
3   ❑ is due to sustained contraction of skeletal muscle

Q57   Stemetil:

1   ❏ is used for labyrinthine disorders
2   ❏ should be used with caution with paracetamol
3   ❏ is available only as a parenteral dosage formulation

Q58   Septicaemia:

1   ❏ occurs when pathogenic microorganisms are present in the blood
2   ❏ is characterised by fever, chills, diarrhoea, nausea and vomiting
3   ❏ is caused only by fungi

Q59   Hypokalaemia:

1   ❏ is characterised by plasma potassium concentration below 60 mmol/l
2   ❏ may be caused by diuretic therapy
3   ❏ is characterised by muscle weakness, cramps

Q60   Patients who complain of abdominal pain should be referred when:

1   ❏ they describe pain as unbearable
2   ❏ it is associated with rapid weight loss
3   ❏ accompanying symptoms include vomiting and constipation

Q61   Infantile seborrhoeic dermatitis:

1   ❏ is one type of eczema
2   ❏ may be relieved by rubbing almond oil before washing the hair
3   ❏ is due to an infection by a microorganism

Q62   Lithium:

1   ❏ is used in the prophylaxis of mania
2   ❏ has a narrow therapeutic index
3   ❏ cannot be used concurrently with diuretics

Q63   Knee caps:

1   ❑ are indicated for soft tissue support
2   ❑ are contraindicated in patients taking NSAIDS
3   ❑ may cause hypersensitivity reactions

Q64   Preparations that could be recommended to a patient who is complaining of dry skin include:

1   ❑ E45 cream
2   ❑ Oilatum bath additive
3   ❑ Nizoral shampoo

Q65   In elderly patients, thyroxine therapy:

1   ❑ is started at a dose of 25 to 50 μg daily
2   ❑ initial dose is adjusted at intervals of at least 4 weeks
3   ❑ a pre-therapy ECG is recommended

Q66   Drugs that may have an adverse effect on contact lens wear include:

1   ❑ Phenergan
2   ❑ Valium
3   ❑ Cilest

Q67   Which of the following drugs do NOT cause dependence?

1   ❑ zolmitriptan
2   ❑ pethidine
3   ❑ morphine

Q68   Neural tube defects are associated with administration during pregnancy of:

1   ❑ phenytoin
2   ❑ carbamazepine
3   ❑ valproate

Q69 A patient comes to the pharmacy requesting Vermox tablets. What advice should be given?

1 ❏ dosage regimen is four times daily for 5 days
2 ❏ Vermox can be used in children under 1 year
3 ❏ all the members of the family should be treated

Q70 A patient comes to the pharmacy requesting advice on a cold. Which of the following symptoms would indicate referral?

1 ❏ rhinorrhoea
2 ❏ dysphagia
3 ❏ pain on coughing

Q71 Cold preparations containing phenylephrine intended for systemic administration should be avoided in patients with:

1 ❏ glaucoma
2 ❏ hypertension
3 ❏ diabetes mellitus

Q72 The laxative action of Duphalac results from:

1 ❏ osmosis
2 ❏ increase in synthesis of prostaglandins
3 ❏ support of growth of colonic bacteria

Q73 Drugs that have a narrow therapeutic index include:

1 ❏ phenytoin
2 ❏ theophylline
3 ❏ codeine

Q74 The advantages of selective serotonin re-uptake inhibitors over the tricyclic antidepressants include:

1 ❏ lower incidence of antimuscarinic side-effects
2 ❏ better effectiveness
3 ❏ less likely to cause gastrointestinal side-effects

Q75 A woman comes to the pharmacy with severe sunburn. Which of the following should be advised?

1 ❏ apply a soothing antiseptic cream
2 ❏ drink plenty of water
3 ❏ apply local anaesthetic

Q76 Dandruff:

1 ❏ is a form of seborrhoeic dermatitis
2 ❏ may indicate the use of Betnovate lotion
3 ❏ suggests the recommendation of shampoos containing coal tar

Q77 Calamine lotion:

1 ❏ has a cooling effect
2 ❏ may be used for chickenpox to promote skin healing
3 ❏ has an emollient effect

Q78 Side-effects that may result in a patient taking 50 mg prednisolone daily for 3 months include:

1 ❏ peptic ulceration
2 ❏ adrenal suppression
3 ❏ subcapsular cataracts

Q79 Sibutramine:

1 ❏ is an opioid drug
2 ❏ inhibits re-uptake of noradrenaline and serotonin
3 ❏ is a centrally acting appetite suppressant

Q80 Back pain may be associated with:

1 ❏ otitis media
2 ❏ osteoporosis
3 ❏ pregnancy

Questions 81–91

Directions: The following questions consist of a first statement followed by a second statement. Decide whether the first statement is true or false. Decide whether the second statement is true or false. Then choose:

A   ❏ if both statements are true and the second statement is a *correct explanation* of the first statement

B   ❏ if both statements are true but the second statement *is NOT a correct explanation* of the first statement

C   ❏ if the first statement is true but the second statement is false

D   ❏ if the first statement is false but the second statement is true

E   ❏ if both statements are false

Directions summarised			
	First statement	**Second statement**	
A	True	True	Second statement is a *correct explanation* of the first
B	True	True	Second statement is *NOT a correct explanation* of the first
C	True	False	
D	False	True	
E	False	False	

Q81   Sirolimus administration requires monitoring of kidney function when given with ciclosporin. Sirolimus has an inhibitory action on the same receptors as ciclosporin.

Q82   Prevenar is a pneumococcal vaccine that contains polysaccharide from seven capsular types of the pneumococcus that is conjugated to protein. Prevenar should only be administered to children who are at an increased risk of pneumococcal infection.

Q83   Patients using Elidel cream should be advised to avoid alcoholic drink during treatment. Elidel may cause folliculitis and impetigo as side-effects.

Q84   In patients with a history of asthma, latanoprost is a preferred first-line treatment in open-angle glaucoma. Latanaprost is available as eye drops and once-daily application in the evening is recommended.

Q85   Patients receiving sorafenib are advised to take tablets with or after food. Sorafenib may cause gastrointestinal disturbances.

Q86   Patients receiving Losec capsules should be advised to swallow the capsule whole. Losec capsules consist of enteric-coated granules, as omeprazole is acid-labile.

Q87   The use of Buscopan tablets is contraindicated in angle-closure glaucoma. Buscopan is a quaternary ammonium compound.

Q88   Bactroban is available as a topical ointment. Bactroban is effective for skin infections caused by Gram-positive organisms.

Q89   Patients taking warfarin should be cautioned not to take medication containing aspirin. Aspirin can cause gastrointestinal bleeding.

Q90   Digital thermometers are safer to use in children than glass thermometers. Digital thermometers are cheaper than glass thermometers.

Q91   Lower initial doses of diuretics should be used in the elderly. The elderly are particularly susceptible to postural hypotension.

Questions 92–100

Directions: These questions involve cases. Read the prescription or case and answer the questions.

Questions 92–94

A 40-year-old male presents with complaints of irritation, skin maceration and malodour in the feet indicating the occurrence of athlete's foot.

Put the following counselling points in order of relevance, assigning 1 to the point that is most relevant and 3 to the point that is least relevant.

Q92   To wash and dry feet thoroughly

Q93   To administer recommended antifungal agent for 10 days after all traces have disappeared

Q94   To use tolnaftate powder as a dusting powder for shoes and socks

Questions 95–97: Use the patient profile below

Patient medication profile

Patient's name: . . . .

Age: 42 years
Allergies: none
Diagnosis: hypertension
Medication history: atenolol 100 mg o.m.
              enalapril maleate 20 mg on
              bendroflumethiazide 5 mg o.m.

The patient comes to the pharmacy complaining of a sudden onset of severe pain in his foot. When the pharmacist examines the patient's foot, the great toe is red and swollen.

Q95   What condition is the patient likely to have?

A   ❑ strain

B   ❑ sprain

C   ❑ arthritis

D   ❑ sting

E   ❑ gout

Q96   Which drug(s) is(are) most likely to be the causative agent of the condition?

1   ❑ bendroflumethiazide

2   ❑ bendroflumethiazide and enalapril

3   ❑ atenolol

A   ❑ 1, 2, 3

B   ❑ 1, 2 only

C   ❑ 2, 3 only

D   ❑ 1 only

E   ❑ 3 only

Q97   Treatment of the condition may be addressed using:

A   ❑ NSAIDs

B   ❑ RICE (rest, ice, compression, elevation) regime

C   ❑ opioid analgesics

D   ❑ corticosteroids

E   ❑ calcitonin

Questions 98–100: Use the prescription below

Patient's name: . . . .

24 years
Ciprofloxacin
250 mg   b.d.   m. 10

Doctor's signature: . . . .

Q98   The patient informs the pharmacist that the physician prescribed the medicine for a urinary tract infection. What non-pharmaceutical advice would you give the patient?

1   ❑ avoid intake of high-fibre foods
2   ❑ increase alcohol intake
3   ❑ increase fluid intake

A   ❑ 1, 2, 3
B   ❑ 1, 2 only
C   ❑ 2, 3 only
D   ❑ 1 only
E   ❑ 3 only

Q99   Ciprofloxacin:

1   ❑ is active against Gram-positive and Gram-negative bacteria
2   ❑ should be used with caution in patients taking NSAIDS
3   ❑ may cause nausea, vomiting, and dyspepsia as side-effects

A   ❑ 1, 2, 3
B   ❑ 1, 2 only
C   ❑ 2, 3 only
D   ❑ 1 only
E   ❑ 3 only

Q100 Urinary tract infections are most commonly caused by:

A   ❑ *Helicobacter pylori*
B   ❑ *Campylobacter jejuni*
C   ❑ *Escherichia coli*
D   ❑ *Mycobacterium tuberculosis*
E   ❑ rhinovirus

Test 3

Answers

A1   B

The refrigerator in the pharmacy intended for the storage of pharmaceutical items should be kept at a temperature of between 2° and 8°C.

A2   D

Fybogel sachets contain ispaghula husk, a bulk-forming laxative, which relieves constipation by increasing the faecal mass through peristalsis. Bulk-forming laxatives are indicated to alleviate constipation in patients with diverticular disease and they could be used on a long-term basis. Patients are also advised to maintain an adequate fluid intake and a diet rich in fibre. Senokot tablets (sennosides), Dulco-lax tablets (bisacodyl) and glycerol suppositories are classified as stimulant laxatives. These increase intestinal motility and must be avoided in intestinal obstruction, such as may occur in diverticular disease. Magnesium hydroxide mixture, which is an osmotic laxative is not indicated in diverticular disease.

A3   D

Sneezing, together with a runny or congested nose and red, itchy eyes, is the most common feature of allergic rhinitis (hay fever). Coloured sputum, fever, sore throat and malaise indicate the presence of an infection, rather than an allergic component.

A4   A

The daily dosing regimen for this patient would be: 25 mg $\times$ 15 kg = 375 mg. Mefenamic acid suspension is available as 50 mg/5 mL. The patient therefore must be given 37.5 mL to receive the total daily dose of 375 mg; 37.5 mL divided into three doses in a day would be equivalent to 12.5 mL. This means that the patient must be given 10 mL on a three times daily (t.d.s.) basis.

A5   C

Co-codamol is a combination of paracetamol (non-opioid analgesic) and codeine (opioid analgesic). One of the side-effects of opioids is constipation. Naprosyn is a proprietary (trade name) preparation of the non-steroidal anti-inflammatory drug naproxen; Adalat is a proprietary preparation of the calcium-channel blocker nifedipine; Amoxil is a proprietary preparation of the beta-lactam amoxicillin; and Dulco-lax is the brand name of the stimulant laxative bisacodyl.

A6   D

Napkin dermatitis can be soothed and prevented with the use of barrier creams and ointments such as zinc and castor oil, Vasogen, Sudocrem and Drapolene. Canesten HC contains an antifungal clotrimazole and the corticosteroid hydrocortisone. Such combination products are only indicated in severe napkin dermatitis and are used only for 1 week, after which treatment is continued with a cream containing an antifungal only.

A7   D

Voltarol is a brand-name preparation for diclofenac (NSAID) and modified-release tablets are available in 75 mg and 100 mg strength. Nu-seals is a proprietary preparation of enteric-coated aspirin 75 mg. Fentanyl, co-codamol and Suboxone (buprenorphine and naloxone) consist of opioid drugs.

A8   A

Amlodipine and nifedipine are dihydropyridine calcium-channel blockers. Amlodipine differs from nifedipine in that it has a longer duration of action and can therefore be given once daily, unlike nifedipine. Both are indicated in hypertension and angina and tend to cause ankle oedema that does not respond to diuretic therapy. Neither amlodipine nor nifedipine are available as spray formulations.

A9 C

Eye infections caused by *Pseudomonas aeruginosa* are associated with severe complications.

A10 C

Gingivitis refers to an inflammation of the gums, which may be caused by poor oral hygiene, dental defects, diabetes and mouth breathing. Gingivitis unlike periodontitis is reversible. Good oral hygiene is encouraged and patients are advised to use an antiseptic mouthwash regularly.

A11 D

Glucose is a simple sugar and is the sole provider of energy to the brain. It is stored in the body as glucagon. Bradykinin, histamine, lymphokines and lysosomal enzymes are all different inflammatory mediators that play a significant role in precipitating asthma and other inflammatory conditions.

A12 E

Staphylococcus aureus, Haemophilus influenzae, Streptococcus pyogenes and *Pseudomonas aeruginosa* are all microorganisms that can cause otitis media. *Enterobius vermicularis* is a threadworm leading to an infection characterised by itchy anus and the presence of white worms.

A13 B

Combined oral contraceptives may cause migraine and are contraindicated in such patients. Progesterone-only contraceptives are more suitable in this case.

A14 C

Ciclosporin, a calcineurin inhibitor, is a potent immunosuppressant useful in the prevention of rejection in organ transplants and grafting procedures. Ciclosporin is markedly nephrotoxic. Vincristine is a vinca alkaloid cytotoxic agent; fluorouracil and methotrexate are both antimetabolite cytotoxic agents; and bleomycin is a cytotoxic antibiotic.

A15   A

Legionnaire's disease is an acute respiratory disease caused by the Gram-negative, aerobic, non-sporing bacillus *Legionella pneumophila*. The disease is transmitted through the inhalation of infected water droplets.

A16   B

Ginvigal hyperplasia is a side-effect commonly associated with phenytoin.

A17   B

The application of a mild topical corticosteroid, such as hydrocortisone, is effective in patients presenting with multiple mosquito bites. Paracetamol, which is an antipyretic agent is not indicated in mosquito bites. Fusidic acid cream is an anti-infective agent and is indicated if the mosquito bites have been scratched and there is risk of infection. Benzocaine (anaesthetic) and mepyramine (antihistamine) may relieve itchiness but are less effective in multiple mosquito bites than hydrocortisone.

A18   A

The difference between ampicillin and amoxicillin is the hydroxyl group that makes amoxicillin more soluble than ampicillin. Amoxicillin is in fact administered three times daily rather than four times daily.

A19   A

Clarithromycin is a macrolide antibacterial agent that should be used with caution in patients with renal impairment. The dose should be reduced if creatinine clearance is less than 30 mL/minute and the modified-release oral preparation should be avoided in this scenario.

A20   C

Co-amoxiclav consists of the combination of amoxicillin (penicillin antibacterial agent) and clavulanic acid (beta-lactamase inhibitor) which is associated with a risk of crystalluria in patients with renal impairment who are receiving high doses, particularly during parenteral therapy.

A21   E

Gentamicin is an aminoglycoside, which is a group of antibacterial agents that is associated with nephrotoxicity and ototoxicity. Their systemic administration to patients with renal impairment should be undertaken carefully but the advantages of this group of antibacterials (particularly their activity against many Gram-negative microorganisms) should outweigh this risk. When gentamicin and other aminoglycosides are used systemically, the serum concentration is monitored to prevent nephrotoxicity and ototoxicity. In patients with renal impairment, drug serum concentration monitoring should be started earlier and more frequent measurements are recommended.

A22   D

Fusidic acid is a narrow-spectrum, antibacterial agent that relies on hepatic elimination. No cautionary action is recommended for patients with renal impairment.

A23   E

Gentamicin, as with other aminoglycosides, is excreted through the kidney, and in renal impairment there is the risk of accumulation. Consequently doses are reduced and dosing interval increased in patients with renal impairment.

A24   A

Metoclopramide is ineffective in motion sickness, as it acts selectively on the chemoreceptor trigger zone. Metoclopramide is effective in treating vomiting associated with gastroduodenal, biliary and hepatic disease, and postoperative vomiting.

A25   B

Promethazine is an antihistamine, which leads to sedation and is therefore used in motion sickness when a sedative effect is desired.

A26   A

Metoclopramide is a dopamine receptor antagonist, which acts selectively on the chemoreceptor trigger zone.

A27   B

Dulco-lax tablets containing bisacodyl, a stimulant laxative, must be swallowed whole with water and not chewed to decrease occurrence of abdominal cramps.

A28   B

Slow-K is a modified-release preparation containing potassium chloride. Patients taking Slow-K are advised to take the tablets in an upright position, while standing or sitting. The tablets should be swallowed whole with plenty of water, to avoid gastrointestinal irritation.

A29   A

Zaditen syrup contains ketotifen, an antihistamine that may cause drowsiness. Patients are therefore advised not to drive or operate machinery.

A30   D

Flagyl tablets contain metronidazole. All patients taking metronidazole are advised to avoid alcohol as the combination of alcohol and metronidazole may lead to a disulfiram-like reaction.

A31   E

Flucloxacillin is a penicillin that must be taken either an hour before food or on an empty stomach for better absorption.

A32   B

Heparin, which has an anticoagulation action, may give rise to heparin-induced thrombocytopenia, which is an immune-mediated condition that usually develops 5–10 days after the administration of the drug. When heparin is used, a platelet count should be measured before treatment and if administration is repeated, platelet counts should be monitored regularly. Signs of thrombocytopenia include a reduction in platelet count. It may present with spontaneous haemorrhage and heparin should be stopped. Factor VIII is used in the treatment and prophylaxis of haemorrhage in patients with haemophilia.

A33   C

Atomoxetine is used in attention deficit hyperactivity disorder (ADHD), which has been associated with a very rare occurrence of hepatic disorders that may present with abdominal pain, unexplained nausea, malaise, darkening of urine or jaundice. Patients and carers are advised to recognise these symptoms and to seek prompt medical attention if they occur. There have been reports of suicidal ideation occurring as a side-effect of atomoxetine therapy. Patients should be advised to report clinical worsening, suicidal thoughts or behaviour, irritability, agitation or depression since these may be signs of development of suicidal ideation. Unlike dexamfetamine, another drug that may be used in ADHD, atomoxetine does not cause tics as a side-effect.

A34   C

Aripiprazole is an atypical antipsychotic agent that is not associated with an impact on prolactin levels and is not associated with impotence as a side-effect. It may precipitate suicidal ideation as a side-effect.

A35   B

Trastuzumab is licensed for the treatment of early breast cancer that overexpresses human epidermal growth factor receptor-2 (HER2). It may be administered as monotherapy or in combination with, for example, paclitaxel, docetaxel (taxanes) or anastrozole (aromatase inhibitors). Since trastuzumab can cause cardiotoxicity, concomitant use with anthracyclines such as doxorubicin should be avoided and requires close monitoring of cardiac function. Trastuzumab is administered by intravenous infusion and may be associated with infusion-related side-effects presenting as chills, fever and hypersensitivity reactions such as anaphylaxis, urticaria and angioedema.

A36   A

Suboxone is a combination of buprenorphine (opioid partial agonist) and naloxone. It is presented as sublingual tablets and is used as an adjunct in the treatment of opioid dependence and in premedication or perioperative analgesia. A side-effect of opioids is drowsiness.

A37   A

Statins should be avoided in active liver disease and unexplained raised serum transaminases. Some antihistamines, such as diphenhydramine and promethazine, should be used with caution in mild-to-moderate liver disease. Selective serotonin re-uptake inhibitors should be used at a reduced dose or avoided in hepatic impairment.

A38   D

Concurrent administration of beta-blockers, such as atenolol, and calcium-channel blockers may result in an enhanced hypotensive effect caused by an additive effect and heart failure may be precipitated.

A39   B

Varilrix is varicella zoster vaccine. All vaccines and Daktacort cream (miconazole and hydrocortisone) must be stored in the refrigerator at a temperature of between 2° and 8°C.

A40   C

Diclofenac is a non-steroidal anti-inflammatory drug. NSAIDs interact with both angiotensin-converting enzyme inhibitors, such as enalapril, and beta-adrenoceptor blockers, such as atenolol, resulting in antagonism to the hypotensive reaction, leading to a hypertensive reaction. NSAIDs interact with diuretics, such as bendroflumethiazide, resulting in an increased risk of nephrotoxicity.

A41   E

Ivabradine is used in the treatment of angina in patients in normal sinus rhythm. It acts on the sinus node resulting in a reduction of the heart rate. It is contraindicated in severe bradycardia (heart rate lower than 60 beats/ minute), cardiogenic shock, acute myocardial infarction, moderate-to-severe heart failure, immediately after a cerebrovascular accident, second and third-degree heart block and patients with unstable angina or a pacemaker. Side-effects include bradycardia, first-degree heart block, ventricular extrasystoles, headache, dizziness and visual disturbances, including blurred vision.

A42   B

Diagnostic testing of body fluids must be carried out in a designated area in the pharmacy. Contaminated waste must be discarded in an appropriate bin.

A43   A

Omeprazole is classified as a proton pump inhibitor, as it acts by blocking the hydrogen–potassium adenosine triphosphate enzyme system of the gastric parietal cells. Omeprazole therefore inhibits gastric acid release. Common side-effects associated with omeprazole include diarrhoea, headache, nausea and vomiting. Concurrent administration of omeprazole and phenytoin results in enhanced effects of phenytoin, which may lead to phenytoin toxicity.

A44   A

Digoxin is a potent positive inotropic cardiac glycoside. Digoxin has a long half-life and the maintenance dose is usually administered once daily. Side-effects, usually associated with overdose, that are characteristic of digoxin toxicity include nausea, vomiting, abdominal pain, diarrhoea and arrhythmias. The geriatric digoxin formulation is available as 62.5 µg tablets.

A45 A

Amiodarone is useful in the treatment of supraventricular and ventricular arrhythmias. Amiodarone tends to have a number of side-effects, such as photosensitivity. Patients are advised to avoid exposure to sunlight and apply a sun protection factor on a daily basis. Amiodarone may also cause reversible corneal microdeposits as a result of which patients find night glare irritating and so patients are advised to avoid driving at night.

A46 A

Simvastatin is a statin. Patients taking statins must be advised to immediately report any unexplained muscle pain, tenderness and weakness and to take the dose preferably at night. Patients must also be advised to follow dietary measures, namely avoid fatty foods and maintain a high-fibre diet.

A47 B

Sumatriptan is a $5HT_1$ (serotonin) agonist indicated in the treatment of migraine. Sumatriptan causes vasoconstriction and must therefore be used with caution in patients with coronary heart disease, such as angina. Concurrent administration of the agonist, sumatriptan and antagonists, such as fluoxetine, which is a selective serotonin re-uptake inhibitor, leads to increased CNS toxicity.

A48 D

Doxycycline, being a tetracycline, is contraindicated in children under 12 years and during pregnancy because tetracyclines tend to be deposited in growing bones and teeth, causing staining and dental hypoplasia. Doxycyline and minocycline are the only tetracyclines that do not exacerbate renal failure and may therefore be administered in patients with renal impairment. Tetracyclines are broad-spectrum antibiotics, active against Gram-negative and Gram-positive microorganisms.

A49   B

Aspirin is avoided in breast-feeding because of the possibility of Reye's syndrome. Moreover if high doses of aspirin are used, the neonate may develop hypoprothrombinaemia. Benzodiazepines such as diazepam are present in milk and therefore should be avoided during breast-feeding. Amoxicillin can be safely administered during pregnancy and breast-feeding.

A50   B

Patients complaining of headache accompanied by nausea, vomiting, nose bleeds, paraesthesia and numbness should be referred.

A51   A

Croup is characterised by a barking cough with high-pitched wheezing that can be heard on expiration. The condition may be accompanied by fever and tachypnoea. Croup is caused by oedema and inflammation of the larynx, epiglottis and vocal cords resulting in narrowing of the airway passages. Croup occurs in babies and young children. It usually occurs at night and may lead to cyanosis and respiratory failure. The condition is rare and requires referral.

A52   A

Verrucas are caused by the human papilloma virus. Verrucas are warts having a characteristic cauliflower-like appearance. Verrucas are contracted from swimming pools and public baths. They are painful when pressure is applied. Treatment involves removal of the hyperkeratolytic skin layers by the use of keratolytic agents such as salicylic acid.

A53   A

Hiatus hernia refers to the protrusion of a portion of the stomach into the thorax through the oesophageal hiatus of the diaphragm. Hiatus hernia is common in obese patients and during pregnancy. Very often the condition is asymptomatic.

A54 D

Coeliac disease refers to a chronic condition in which the small intestine has an unusual sensitivity to gluten. The condition may be secondary to lactose intolerance. Patients with coeliac disease must therefore follow a gluten-free diet.

A55 A

Chilblains are areas of the skin that are locally inflamed and bluish-red in colour. They occur as a reaction to cold, damp weather. The lesions are very often accompanied by tenderness and intense pruritus.

A56 B

Migraine headache may be triggered by a variety of factors, including chocolate. Patients are advised to try and identify triggering factors, to avoid migraine attacks as much as possible. Migraine attacks may or may not be preceded by an aura consisting of visual disturbances, blind spots or flashing lights. The aetiology of migraine is unknown. Sustained contraction of the skeletal muscle is associated with tension headache and not with migraine headache.

A57 D

Stemetil is a proprietary preparation of prochlorperazine, a phenothiazine used in vertigo and labyrinthine disorders. Stemetil is available as tablets, syrup and injection. There is no contraindication to the concurrent use of paracetamol and prochlorperazine.

A58 B

Septicaemia occurs when pathogenic microorganisms or their toxins are present in the bloodstream. Septicaemia is a serious condition characterised by fever, chills, diarrhoea, nausea and vomiting.

A59   C

Hypokalaemia occurs when the plasma-potassium level falls below 3.0 mmol/L. Hypokalaemia may occur following loop or thiazide diuretic therapy. Patients at risk of developing hypokalaemia are often prescribed potassium supplements to counteract the potassium loss caused by the diuretic therapy. Symptoms of hypokalaemia include muscle weakness and cramps. . Severe cases may lead to muscle paralysis and respiratory failure.

A60   A

Abdominal pain accompanied by rapid weight loss, vomiting and constipation, and which is unbearable in nature requires referral to exclude peptic ulcers, diverticular disease and carcinoma.

A61   B

Infantile seborrhoeic dermatitis or cradle cap, is a type of eczema common in infants. It presents as scaling and crusting of the scalp within the first three months of life and resolves spontaneously within a year. Management of the condition includes the application and rubbing of almond oil, baby oil, olive oil or clove oil into the scalp, leaving the oil overnight and then washing it off the following day.

A62   A

Lithium is a drug with a narrow therapeutic index and therefore plasma concentrations are regularly monitored. Lithium is used in the prophylaxis and treatment of mania. Concurrent administration of lithium and diuretics, particularly the thiazides, is contraindicated as lithium excretion is reduced, resulting in increased plasma-lithium concentration and hence toxicity.

A63   D

Knee caps, which are indicated for soft tissue support, are not contraindicated in patients taking non-steroidal anti-inflammatory drugs. Knee caps do not result in hypersensitivity reactions.

A64   B

Oilatum bath additive and E45 cream are both emollients that soothe, smooth and hydrate the skin, so are useful in dry skin conditions. Nizoral shampoo is an antifungal preparation containing ketoconazole that is used in dandruff.

A65   A

Thyroxine is used in hypothyroidism, a condition that may well present in elderly patients. Side-effects of thyroxine usually occur at excessive doses and include gastrointestinal disturbances (nausea, vomiting) as well as cardiac symptoms such as angina pain, arrhythmias, palpitation and tachycardia. Thyroxine should be used with caution in elderly patients as they are more prone to side-effects. A lower initial dose (25–50 µg daily) is recommended for patients who are over 50 years. Dose adjustments should take place at intervals of at least 4 weeks. A pretreatment electrocardiogram is recommended because changes induced by hypothyroidism (that would be present at baseline) may be confused with ischaemia.

A66   A

Phenergan contains the antihistamine promethazine. Valium contains the benzodiazepine diazepam. Both the antihistamine and the benzodiazepine tend to reduce the blink rate, leading to dry eyes. Cilest is a combined oral contraceptive, which, like other oral contraceptives, may cause reduced tolerance because of corneal and eyelid oedema.

A67   D

Pethidine and morphine, used as opioid analgesics, may cause dependence following repeated administration. Zolmitriptan, a $5HT_1$ agonist used in the treatment of acute migraine attacks, is not associated with dependence.

A68   A

Anti-epileptic drugs, such as phenytoin, carbamazepine and valproate, may lead to neural tube defects if administered during pregnancy. Concurrent administration of folate supplements, such as folic acid, is recommended.

A69   E

Vermox is a proprietary preparation of mebendazole, an anthelmintic drug indicated for threadworm or ringworm infections. Mebendazole is administered as a single dose. A second dose can be administered 2–3 weeks after the first dose to prevent re-infection. All members of the family must be treated if the infection is detected in one family member. Use of mebendazole in children under 2 years is not recommended.

A70   C

Patients presenting at the pharmacy complaining of common cold accompanied by pain on coughing and dysphagia warrant referral.

A71   A

Phenylephrine is a nasal decongestant that mimics the sympathetic system, thereby increasing the heart rate and blood pressure. It may aggravate conditions such as diabetes, hypertension and glaucoma. Patients with hypertension, ischaemic heart disease, hyperthyroidism, diabetes and glaucoma are therefore given topical nasal sympathomimetics rather than systemic sympathomimetics. Both topical and systemic sympathomimetics are contraindicated in patients taking monoamine oxidase inhibitors, because concurrent administration of the two products may lead to a hypertensive crisis.

A72   D

Duphalac is a proprietary preparation of lactulose, an osmotic laxative. Lactulose, which is a semi-synthetic disaccharide, is not absorbed from the gastrointestinal tract and produces an osmotic diarrhoea of low faecal pH, which discourages the proliferation of ammonia-producing organisms.

A73   B

Both phenytoin and theophylline have a narrow therapeutic index.

A74   D

Selective serotonin re-uptake inhibitors such as paroxetine tend to cause less antimuscarinic side-effects and are less toxic in overdose than the tricylic antidepressants, such as amitriptyline. However, selective serotonin re-uptake inhibitors are more likely to cause gastrointestinal disturbances, such as nausea and vomiting, than tricylic antidepressants. Selective serotonin re-uptake inhibitors and tricylic antidepressants are equally effective.

A75   B

The application of a soothing antiseptic cream is the first-choice treatment in patients complaining of severe sunburn. Patients are advised to drink a lot of water to avoid getting dehydrated. A cold shower before going to bed makes the patient feel more comfortable. The application of a local anaesthetic may cause hypersensitivity and is only addressing the pain issue.

A76   A

Dandruff is a form of seborrhoeic dermatitis. Management of dandruff lies with the application of a mild detergent shampoo once or twice a week. Shampoos containing coal tar may be recommended; however, the use of such shampoos is not first-line treatment. Betnovate lotion containing betamethasone, a potent corticosteroid, may be useful in severe dandruff.

A77   B

Calamine lotion is mildly astringent, soothing and has a cooling effect. It is therefore useful in itchy skin conditions, such as chickenpox.

A78   A

Long-term use of oral corticosteroids may result in side-effects, such as peptic ulceration, adrenal suppression and subcapsular cataracts.

A79 C

Sibutramine is a centrally acting appetite suppressant used as an adjunct in the management of obesity. It inhibits the re-uptake of noradrenaline and serotonin.

A80 C

Otitis media is inflammation or infection of the middle ear and is not usually associated with back pain. Osteoporosis is a condition occurring mostly in postmenopausal women and is characterised by brittle bones caused by reduced bone mass. It is presented with pain. If it occurs in the vertebral structure the condition may be associated with chronic back pain. Pregnancy may be associated with back pain because of an increase in weight and the increased strain.

A81 C

Sirolimus is a calcineurin inhibitor that acts as an immunosuppressant. It is administered systemically in the prophylaxis of organ rejection in kidney allograft recipients. It may be used in combination with ciclosporin, particularly initially. However since ciclosporin is markedly nephrotoxic, when sirolimus is used with ciclosporin, monitoring of kidney function is essential.

A82 C

Prevenar is the pneumococcal polysaccharide-conjugate vaccine and contains polysaccharide, from seven capsular types of pneumococci, which is conjugated to diphtheria toxin (protein). Prevenar is recommended for individuals at increased risk of pneumococcal infection including those over 65 years, patients with chronic heart, renal, respiratory or liver disease, diabetics and immune deficiency. It is a component of the primary course of childhood immunisation.

A83   B

Elidel cream consists of pimecrolimus, which is a calcineurin inhibitor that is used for eczema or psoriasis. Patients should be advised to avoid alcoholic drink during the treatment period as consumption of alcohol may lead to facial flushing and skin irritation. Side-effects associated with the topical administration of pimecrolimus include a burning sensation, pruritus, erythema and skin infections, including folliculitis and, less commonly, impetigo.

A84   B

Latanoprost is a prostaglandin analogue that is available for topical administration in raised intraocular pressure in open-angle glaucoma. Since topical administration of beta-blockers such as timolol is not recommended in patients with asthma because of the risk of inducing bronchospasm, prostaglandin analogues are usually the preferred first-line treatment. Latanoprost should be applied once daily in the evening.

A85   D

Sorafenib is a protein kinase inhibitor that is used in malignant disease. Patients should be advised to take tablets an hour before food or on an empty stomach. Side-effects include gastrointestinal disturbances including diarrhoea or constipation, dyspepsia, dysphagia and anorexia.

A86   A

Losec consists of omeprazole, a proton pump inhibitor. Proton pump inhibitors are acid-labile. Losec consists of enteric-coated granules that are encapsulated. Patients are advised to swallow the capsule whole.

A87   B

Buscopan is a branded preparation containing hyoscine butylbromide, an antimuscarinic agent that reduces gastrointestinal motility. Antimuscarinic agents are contraindicated in cases of angle-closure glaucoma as they may aggrevate the condition. Hyoscine butylbromide is a quaternary ammonium compound, unlike atropine, which is a tertiary ammonium compound.

Quaternary ammonium compounds are less lipid-soluble and therefore tend to cause fewer central atropine-like side-effects, whereas peripheral side-effects are more common.

A88   B

Bactroban is the trade name for the topical preparation containing mupirocin. Bactroban is available as nasal ointment or skin ointment. Mupirocin is very effective for treating skin infections caused by Gram-positive organisms but it is not active against Gram-negative microorganisms. Mupirocin should not be used for longer than 10 days, to avoid development of resistance.

A89   A

Warfarin is an oral anticoagulant. Aspirin may cause gastrointestinal bleeding through its cyclo-oxygenase-1 interference. The concomittant administration of warfarin and aspirin potentiates the risk of bleeding; moreover, internal haemorrhage is very dangerous.

A90   C

Digital thermometers are safer to use in children than glass thermometers as there is no risk of the glass being broken. Digital thermometers tend to be more expensive.

A91   A

Elderly patients must be started on the lowest possible dose of diuretics as they tend to be more susceptible to their side-effects, such as postural hypotension.

A92–94

The use of topical antifungal agents (imidazole antifungals and terbinafine) is the first-line of treatment in athlete's foot. Patients should be advised to be persistent in treatment and that application of the product should be continued for about 10 days after all traces have disappeared. This will ensure eradication. Patient should be educated on non-pharmacotherapeutic measures and adjunctive therapy that contribute towards the management of the condition. The area should be washed regularly and dried thoroughly as fungal infection predominates in moist environments. The use of tolnaftate powder as a dusting powder for shoes and socks limits re-infection from contaminated footwear. The powder also acts as a moisture adsorbent.

A92   2

A93   1

A94   3

A95   E

Diuretics such as bendroflumethiazide tend to cause gout, a condition characterised by a red, swollen great toe caused by the deposition of uric acid at the metatarsophalangeal joint.

A96   D

Gout is a common side-effect of diuretics such as bendroflumethiazide.

A97   A

Management of an acute attack of gout involves the use of high doses of non-steroidal anti-inflammatory agents (NSAIDs). Colchicine is useful in patients with heart failure where the use of NSAIDs is contraindicated because of water retention. Allopurinol and other uricosuric agents are not indicated for acute attacks as they may aggravate the condition. The use of an intra-articular corticosteroid injection in gout is unlicensed.

A98   E

Increasing fluid intake would help flush out urinary tract infections.

A99   A

Ciprofloxacin is a quinolone active against both Gram-positive and Gram-negative organisms. All quinolones must be used with caution in patients taking non-steroidal anti-inflammatory agents as the concurrent administration of the two agents may lead to convulsions. Common side-effects of quinolones include nausea, vomiting and dyspepsia.

A100   C

Urinary tract infections are very commonly caused by Gram-negative bacteria such as *Escherichia coli*, the *Proteus* species and *Pseudomonas* species.

Test 4

Questions

Questions 1–5

Directions: Each of the questions or incomplete statements is followed by five suggested answers. Select the best answer in each case.

Q1   The Summaries of Product Characteristics (SPCs):

   A   ❑ are issued by a medicines regulatory agency
   B   ❑ have to be updated every year
   C   ❑ are intended for patients' use
   D   ❑ are the same for generic formulations as for the originator products
   E   ❑ reflect information in the marketing authorisations of medicinal products

Q2   Unlicensed use of a medicine applies to:

   A   ❑ changing an adult oral dosage form to a liquid formulation for administration to a paediatric patient
   B   ❑ use of a generic formulation instead of the originator product
   C   ❑ a request to the manufacturer for a specific amount of product for a one-time use
   D   ❑ the use of therapeutically equivalent licensed products
   E   ❑ the use of a product that is licensed with EMEA

Q3 Suspected adverse reactions:

A ❑ are reported by health professionals directly to the European medicines agency

B ❑ may be reported only by pharmacists

C ❑ to any therapeutic agent should be reported

D ❑ should be immediately disseminated to the media to alert the public

E ❑ should be investigated by the regulatory body and, if necessary, the drug should be withdrawn prior to informing the marketing authorisation holder

Q4 Methadone:

A ❑ has a long duration of action

B ❑ is only available for parenteral administration

C ❑ is an opioid antagonist

D ❑ is not addictive

E ❑ does not present the risk of toxicity in non-opioid dependent adults

Q5 The following statements are all applicable for a community pharmacy EXCEPT:

A ❑ premises are easily accessible to the public

B ❑ walls, floors, ceilings and windows are kept clean in such manner that any surfaces present shall be impervious and may be easily wiped clean

C ❑ the premises have a clear area set aside for the preparation and compounding of medicinal products and diagnostic testing

D ❑ all pharmaceutical and non-pharmaceutical waste and expired and deteriorated products are to be segregated from pharmacy stock

E ❑ shop window is unobstructed when the pharmacy is closed to ensure that external appearance reflects the professional character of the pharmacy

Questions 6–15

Directions: Each group of questions below consists of five lettered headings followed by a list of numbered questions. For each numbered question select the one heading that is most closely related to it. Each heading may be used once, more than once, or not at all.

Questions 6–10 concern the use of the following drugs during pregnancy:

A   ❑ co-trimoxazole
B   ❑ gliclazide
C   ❑ mesalazine
D   ❑ lisinopril
E   ❑ streptomycin

Select, from A to E, which one of the above:

Q6   may cause skull defects

Q7   has an increased risk of neonatal haemolysis during the third trimester

Q8   may cause vestibular or auditory nerve damage

Q9   should be stopped at least 2 days before delivery

Q10   consists of a folate antagonist that poses a teratogenic risk

Questions 11–15 concern the following products:

A   ❏ Bezalip
B   ❏ Ezetrol
C   ❏ Lescol XL
D   ❏ Questran
E   ❏ Zocor

Select, from A to E, which one of the above:

Q11   inhibits the intestinal absorption of cholesterol

Q12   acts mainly by decreasing serum triglycerides

Q13   is used in pruritus associated with partial biliary obstruction

Q14   is an anion-exchange resin

Q15   is a modified-release formulation

Questions 16–49

Directions: For each of the questions below, ONE or MORE of the
responses is (are) correct. Decide which of the responses is
(are) correct. Then choose

A   ❏ if 1, 2 and 3 are correct
B   ❏ if 1 and 2 only are correct
C   ❏ if 2 and 3 only are correct
D   ❏ if 1 only is correct
E   ❏ if 3 only is correct

Directions summarised				
A	**B**	**C**	**D**	**E**
1, 2, 3	1, 2 only	2, 3 only	1 only	3 only

Q16   Sitagliptin:

1   ❏ decreases insulin secretion
2   ❏ should not be used with metformin
3   ❏ may cause hypoglycaemia as a side-effect

Q17   Lucentis:

1   ❏ is a vascular endothelial growth factor inhibitor
2   ❏ is administered by intravitreal injection
3   ❏ requires activation by local irradiation using non-thermal red light

Q18   In juvenile chronic arthritis:

1   ❏ inflammatory joint disease occurs before 16 years of age
2   ❏ ibuprofen may be used at a dose of 30–40 mg/kg (maximum 2.4 g) daily
3   ❏ diclofenac is not recommended in children under 16 years of age

Q19   Babies:

1   ❏ under 6 months of age who have a temperature higher than 37.7°C should be referred to see a doctor on the same day
2   ❏ who had a prolonged, temperature-related convulsion lasting 15 minutes or longer may be treated with diazepam, preferably rectally in solution
3   ❏ long-term anticonvulsant prophylaxis for febrile convulsions is rarely indicated

Q20   Acute laryngotracheobronchitis:

1   ❏ usually occurs as a result of narrowing of the airway in the region of the larynx

2   ❏ dexamethasone 150 μg/kg as a single dose may be used

3   ❏ in severe cases nebulised adrenaline (epinephrine) solution may be considered

Q21   The risk of conceiving a child with a neural tube defect is:

1   ❏ increased by using folic acid at a dose of 4 μg/day

2   ❏ increased in women taking lamotrigine

3   ❏ increased in women with diabetes mellitus

Q22   Exelon patches:

1   ❏ patients who are taking 9 mg orally of Exelon daily and who are not tolerating the dose well may be shifted to the transdermal patch using 4.6 mg/24 hours, applying the first patch on the day after the last oral dose

2   ❏ same sites of application should not be re-used within 14 days

3   ❏ patient's body weight should be monitored during treatment

Q23   Rasilez:

1   ❏ should be used with caution if estimated glomerular filtration rate is less than 80 mL/minute

2   ❏ should not be used in patients taking other antihypertensives

3   ❏ tablets should be taken with or after food

Q24   Trabectedin:

1   ❏ does not cause gastrointestinal side-effects

2   ❏ requires monitoring of hepatic parameters

3   ❏ requires the concomitant intravenous infusion of dexamethasone

Q25 Cerebral oedema:

1 ❑ may present with pupillary vasoconstriction
2 ❑ is treated with mannitol by intravenous infusion at a dose of 200 g/kg as a 15–20% solution
3 ❑ may result from hypoxia at high altitude

Q26 Use of fluvoxamine in obsessive-compulsive disorder:

1 ❑ in children over 8 years is started at 25 mg daily
2 ❑ should be reconsidered if no improvement occurs within 10 weeks
3 ❑ may be administered with an MAOI

Q27 Somatomedins:

1 ❑ are a group of polypeptide hormones structurally related to insulin
2 ❑ should be used with caution in patients with diabetes
3 ❑ may induce bradycardia

Q28 In patients with cancer the use of erythropoietins:

1 ❑ may increase the risk of thrombosis
2 ❑ is intended to shorten the period of symptomatic anaemia in patients with cancer not receiving chemotherapy
3 ❑ is administered to achieve a target haemoglobin concentration higher than 12 g/100 mL

Q29 Pegzerepoetin alfa:

1 ❑ has a longer duration of action than epoetin
2 ❑ may be administered by subcutaneous injection
3 ❑ should not be used in chronic kidney disease

Q30   In patients receiving long-term warfarin who undergo a dental extraction:

1   ❑ an INR assessment should be carried out 72 hours before the procedure

2   ❑ warfarin may be continued in patients with an INR below 4.0 without dose adjustments

3   ❑ metronidazole therapy may enhance effect of warfarin

Q31   In anaphylaxis, adrenaline (epinephrine) administration:

1   ❑ is preferably carried out by the intramuscular route

2   ❑ requires monitoring of blood pressure, pulse and respiratory function

3   ❑ may be followed by a slow intravenous injection of chlorphenamine

Q32   Rhabdomyolysis may occur as a side-effect of:

1   ❑ nicotinic acid

2   ❑ aripiprazole

3   ❑ propofol

Q33   Concomitant use of Tegretol should be avoided with:

1   ❑ ranitidine

2   ❑ gabapentin

3   ❑ clarithromycin

Q34   Which of the following preparations may be administered in the ear?:

1   ❑ Sofradex

2   ❑ Canesten

3   ❑ Nasonex

Q35 Clinically significant drug interactions with ciclosporin could occur with:

1 ❑ Coversyl
2 ❑ Ciproxin
3 ❑ Tenormin

Q36 Malaria:

1 ❑ is transmitted by the bite from the female *Anopheles* mosquito
2 ❑ has an incubation period of up to 10 days
3 ❑ is widespread in Australia

Q37 In malaria, standby medication:

1 ❑ refers to a course of self-administered antimalarial treatment for use by travellers visiting remote malarious areas
2 ❑ is used if fever of 38°C or more develops 7 days or more after leaving a malarious area
3 ❑ consists of drugs that have been used for chemoprophylaxis by the traveller

Q38 Chemoprophylaxis of malaria with mefloquine can be undertaken with caution in:

1 ❑ pregnancy
2 ❑ epilepsy
3 ❑ cardiac conduction disorders

Q39 *Pneumocystis carinii* pneumonia:

1 ❑ is associated with immunocompromised patients
2 ❑ may be treated with co-trimoxazole
3 ❑ is rarely fatal if untreated

Q40   Pompholyx:

1   ❑ often affects the hands and feet
2   ❑ presents with pruritus
3   ❑ is contagious

Q41   Arnica:

1   ❑ is traditionally used for sprains and bruises
2   ❑ contains terpenoids
3   ❑ is not suitable for internal use

Q42   Genital warts:

1   ❑ present an average incubation period of 2–3 months
2   ❑ may become more widespread during pregnancy
3   ❑ are associated with the possibility of relapse in some patients

Q43   Imiquimod cream:

1   ❑ is used only for soft, non-keratinised lesions
2   ❑ may cause local ulceration
3   ❑ is rubbed in the area and should be washed off with mild
soap and water after a specified time

Q44   Silver nitrate:

1   ❑ is a caustic agent
2   ❑ is presented as a stick or pencil in combination with potassium nitrate
3   ❑ may stain skin and fabric

Q45   Tetracosactide:

1   ❑ is an analogue of corticotropin
2   ❑ may be used as a diagnostic test administered by intramuscular injection
3   ❑ may be used in the treatment of fertility

Q46   Huntington's chorea:

1   ❑ is associated with rheumatic fever
2   ❑ has an insidious onset and usually occurs in early adulthood
3   ❑ affects personality and commonly presents with severe depression

Q47   Disadvantages of using tetrabenazine in Huntington's chorea are:

1   ❑ depletion of nerve endings of dopamine
2   ❑ effectiveness in only a proportion of patients
3   ❑ occurrence of depression as a side-effect

Q48   Whipple's disease:

1   ❑ is caused by a bacterial infection of the small intestine
2   ❑ symptoms are restricted to the gastrointestinal tract
3   ❑ treatment relies on antidiarrhoeal agents

Q49   Gelatin intravenous infusion:

1   ❑ is preferred to albumin in burns
2   ❑ requires adjustment of fluid and electrolyte therapy at all times
3   ❑ requires monitoring of urine output

Questions 50–80

Directions: The following questions consist of a first statement followed by a second statement. Decide whether the first statement is true or false. Decide whether the second statement is true or false. Then choose:

A ❏ if both statements are true and the second statement is a *correct explanation* of the first statement

B ❏ if both statements are true but the second statement *is NOT a correct explanation* of the first statement

C ❏ if the first statement is true but the second statement is false

D ❏ if the first statement is false but the second statement is true

E ❏ if both statements are false

Directions summarised			
	First statement	**Second statement**	
A	True	True	Second statement is a *correct explanation* of the first
B	True	True	Second statement is *NOT a correct explanation* of the first
C	True	False	
D	False	True	
E	False	False	

Q50 Intravenous midazolam is often preferred to intravenous diazepam as a sedative in combined anaesthesia. Midazolam is water-soluble and recovery is faster than from diazepam.

Q51 Infliximab is administered by subcutaneous injection at an initial dose of 5 mg/kg repeated after 2 weeks. Infliximab may be used as maintenance therapy in patients with Crohn's disease who responded to the initial induction course.

Q52 Glyceryl trinitrate may be used topically every 12 hours for anal fissures. Glyceryl trinitrate is a nitrovasodilator that causes the anal sphincter to relax when applied topically.

Q53 Before initiating treatment with omalizumab, body weight and immunoglobulin E concentration need to be determined. Omalizumab is a monoclonal antibody administered by subcutaneous injection for the prophylaxis of allergic asthma.

Q54 Baseline prothrombin time should be measured in patients receiving abciximab. Abciximab is an antiplatelet agent that acts by increasing the binding of fibrinogen to receptors on platelets.

Q55 Avandia is useful when there is failing insulin release. Avandia reduces peripheral insulin resistance.

Q56 Avandia treatment should be started in combination with insulin. Blood-glucose control may deteriorate temporarily when Avandia is substituted for an oral antidiabetic drug.

Q57 Dexamethasone oral therapy is preferred during pregnancy to prednisolone. Dexamethasone is a fluorinated corticosteroid that does not cross the placenta readily.

Q58 Patients receiving bupropion should avoid using promethazine. Bupropion causes sedation as a side-effect.

Q59 Cigarette smoking should stop completely before starting varenicline. Varenicline may cause dry mouth, taste disturbance and aphthous stomatitis as side-effects.

Q60 Tibolone is preferred to continuous combined HRT preparations in premenopausal women. Tibolone poses an increased risk of thromboembolism compared with combined HRT or women not taking HRT.

Q61 Patients receiving Bonviva 150 mg tablets for the treatment of postmenopausal osteoporosis are advised to take one tablet once a month. Patients should be advised to take the Bonviva 150 mg tablet at least 1 hour before breakfast or another oral medicine.

Q62 Before the patient is started on Actonel, preventive dental treatment should be considered. Actonel is associated with osteonecrosis of the jaw.

Q63 In patients receiving bevacizumab, parameters that should be monitored include blood pressure. Bevacizumab may cause congestive heart failure as a side-effect.

Q64 The dose of allopurinol should be reduced in patients receiving azathioprine. Both allopurinol and azathioprine may cause hypersensitivity reactions.

Q65 Daunorubicin should be diluted with infusion fluid to a concentration of 1mg/mL and given over 20 minutes. Daunorubicin is an anthracycline antibiotic that is highly irritant to tissues.

Q66 Methotrexate should be avoided in a patient with a creatinine clearance of 12 mL/minute. Methotrexate is an antimetabolite drug that is nephrotoxic.

Q67 When habitual abortion is due to incompetence of the cervix, suturing of the cervix may be adopted. Dydrogesterone is recommended as a first-line treatment in patients with a history of recurrent miscarriage.

Q68 Severe pain in one loin, which may last several hours and recur at intervals of days requires referral. The patient needs to be assessed for the occurrence of renal calculi.

Q69 Urinary retention may occur with the use of trimipramine. Trimipramine has antimuscarinic activity.

Q70 Lithium should be stopped 24 hours before major surgery. Lithium should be avoided if possible in renal impairment.

Q71 In patients suffering from Addison's disease, lithium should be used with caution. Addison's disease is associated with sodium imbalance.

Q72   In anaesthesia, nitrous oxide may be used up to a concentration of 66% in oxygen. Nitrous oxide is unsatisfactory as a sole anaesthetic.

Q73   Desflurane is preferred to isoflurane for induction of anaesthesia because it is rapid acting. Desflurane is a liquid at room temperature.

Q74   Prilocaine should be avoided in patients receiving co-amoxiclav. Prilocaine may cause ocular toxicity when used for ophthalmic procedures.

Q75   Cocaine causes agitation, tachycardia and hypertension. Cocaine stimulates the central nervous system.

Q76   Lantus may be considered in type II diabetic patients whose lifestyle is severely restricted by recurrent symptomatic hypoglycaemia. Lantus should not be used in combination with metformin.

Q77   Giant cell arteritis may present with tender and non-pulsatile temporal arteries together with erythema and oedema of the overlying skin. The condition may require the use of prednisolone tablets for at least 2 years.

Q78   Flecainide can precipitate serious arrhythmias only in patients with a history of myocardial infarction. Flecainide is a membrane stabilising drug.

Q79   As opposed to flecainide, amiodarone is not associated with pneumonitis as a side-effect. Signs of pneumonitis include progressive shortness of breath or cough.

Q80   Disulfiram should not be used in patients with a history of cerebrovascular accidents. Disulfiram may cause peripheral neuritis as a side-effect.

Questions 81–100

Directions: Read the patient request and follow the instructions.

Questions 81–85: For the following products, place your order of preference for a preparation to be used in severe onychomycosis in a toenail. Assign 1 to the product that should be recommended as first choice and 5 to the product that should be least recommended.

Q81   Daktarin cream twice daily for 3 months

Q82   Lamisil tablets 250 mg daily for 3 months

Q83   Nizoral cream once daily for 3 months

Q84   Sporanox capsules 200 mg twice daily for 7 days

  repeated after 21 day interval for three courses

Q85   Zovirax cream twice daily for 1 month

Questions 86–89: Put the following side-effects of mirtazapine in order of probability of occurrence, assigning 1 to the most frequent side-effect and 4 to the least common side-effect.

Q86   abnormal dreams

Q87   angle-closure glaucoma

Q88   dizziness

Q89   sedation

Questions 90–92:

A patient who is taking phenytoin and is hypersensitive to penicillin requires a broad-spectrum antibacterial agent for a respiratory tract infection.

For the following products, place your order of preference, assigning 1 to the product that should be recommended as first choice and 3 to the product that should be recommended as a last choice.

Q90   Ciproxin

Q91   Flagyl

Q92   Zithromax

Questions 93–97:

A patient presents with a prescription for cefalexin capsules. The product is not available. An alternative preparation needs to be discussed with the prescriber.

For the following products, place your order of preference, assigning 1 to the product that should be recommended as first choice and 5 to the product that should be recommended as a last choice.

Q93   Augmentin tablets

Q94   Klaricid tablets

Q95   Rocephin injections

Q96   Utinor tablets

Q97   Zinnat tablets

Questions 98–100:

A patient presents with mild-to-moderate acne.

For the following products, place your order of preference, assigning 1 to the product that should be recommended as first choice and 3 to the product that should be recommended as a last choice.

Q98   Dalacin capsules

Q99   Panoxyl gel

Q100 Roaccutane capsules

Test 4

Answers

A1   E

The Summary of Product Characteristics (SPC) for a medicinal product reflects the information in the marketing authorisation of the product. It is prepared by the manufacturer and is intended for health professionals. Updates are necessary to reflect any approved changes by the regulatory body in the marketing authorisation.

A2   A

An example of a scenario when a medicine use is unlicensed is when an adult oral dosage form is changed to a liquid formulation for administration to a paediatric patient.

A3   C

When health professionals (doctors, dentists, pharmacists, nurses) suspect an adverse reaction to any therapeutic agent including drugs, blood products, vaccines, radiographic contrast media, complementary and herbal products, they should follow the process established by the national regulatory agency. In the United Kingdom, the Medicines and Healthcare products Regulatory Agency (MHRA) has the Yellow Card Scheme through which health professionals can report suspected adverse reactions either by completing the card or electronically.

A4   A

Methadone is an opioid analgesic that is available for oral and parenteral administration. It is used in severe pain, in palliative care and as an adjunct in the management of opioid dependence. Compared with morphine, it is less sedating and has a longer duration of action. It may lead to addiction and can still cause toxicity when used in adults with non-opioid dependency. Because of the long duration of action, in overdosage, patients need to be monitored for long periods.

A5   E

Community pharmacies should be easily accessible to the public and maintained in a clean condition. Walls, floors, ceilings and windows must be kept clean and surfaces should be impervious and easily wiped. The premises should have a clear area set aside for the preparation and compounding of medicinal products and diagnostic testing, and all pharmaceutical or non-pharmaceutical waste and expired or deteriorated items should be segregated in a separate area. When the pharmacy is closed, the shop window may be totally closed off with aluminium shutters for security purposes.

A6   D

Lisinopril is an angiotensin-converting enzyme (ACE) inhibitor and ACE inhibitors should be avoided during pregnancy. ACE inhibitors may adversely affect fetal and neonatal blood pressure control and renal function. They may also cause neonatal skull defects.

A7   A

Co-trimoxazole is a folate antagonist and should be avoided in the first and the third trimesters of pregnancy. In the third trimester there is an increased risk of neonatal haemolysis and methaemoglobinaemia, whereas in the first trimester there is a teratogenic risk caused by the trimethoprim (folate antagonist) component.

A8   E

All aminoglycosides are associated with auditory or vestibular nerve damage, especially during the second and third trimesters. The risk is greatest with streptomycin and is lower with gentamicin and tobramycin.

A9   B

Gliclazide is a sulphonylurea. In general, diabetic patients are switched over to insulin during pregnancy. Sulphonylureas should be stopped at least 2 days before delivery (in patients who are still receiving them) because of the risk of neonatal hypoglycaemia.

A10   A

Co-trimoxazole consists of trimethoprim and sulphamethoxazole combined because of their synergistic antimicrobial effects. Trimethoprim is a folate antagonist that poses a teratogenic risk.

A11   B

Ezetrol contains ezetimibe, which selectively inhibits absorption of cholesterol in the intestine. It is used as monotherapy or in combination with other drug therapy as an adjunct to lifestyle measures in patients with hypercholesterolaemia.

A12   A

Bezalip is bezafibrate that, being a fibrate, acts mainly by decreasing serum triglycerides. Fibrates have variable effects on low-density-lipoprotein cholesterol.

A13   D

Questran contains colestyramine, a lipid-regulating drug that acts as a bile acid sequestrant; it is also used in pruritus associated with partial biliary obstruction and primary biliary cirrhosis.

A14   D

Questran, which is colestyramine, binds to bile acids resulting in prevention of their re-absorption and hence promoting hepatic conversion of cholesterol into bile acids.

A15   C

Lescol XL, is a modified-release preparation of fluvastatin 80 mg, a statin.

A16   E

Sitagliptin is a dipeptidylpeptidase-4 inhibitor that increases insulin secretion and lowers glucagon secretion. Sitagliptin is available for oral administration. It is indicated in patients with type 2 diabetes mellitus in combination with either metformin (biguanide) or a sulphonylurea or a thiazolidinedione.

A17   B

Lucentis contains ranibizumab and is available for intravitreal injection. It is a vascular endothelial growth factor inhibitor indicated for the treatment of neovascular (wet) age-related macular degeneration. Unlike verteporfin, which is used in photodynamic treatment of age-related macular degeneration, ranibizumab does not require activation by local irradiation using non-thermal red light.

A18   B

Juvenile chronic arthritis is defined as a group of systemic inflammatory disorders affecting children below the age of 16 years. Pharmacotherapy is aimed to reduce pain and non-steroidal anti-inflammatory drugs are used. Ibuprofen is used at a dose of 30–40 mg/kg daily up to a maximum of 2.4 g. Other agents used include diclofenac at a dose of 1–3 mg/kg daily.

A19   A

The normal body temperature is 36.8°C. Babies under 6 months of age who have a higher temperature than 37.7°C should be referred on the same day. Babies over 6 months should be referred if their temperature is above 38.2°C. Babies who have had a temperature-related convulsion lasting 15 minutes or longer should receive pharmacotherapy in the form of either lorazepam, diazepam or clonazepam. Febrile convulsions in children usually cease spontaneously within 5–10 minutes and are rarely associated with significant sequelae and therefore long-term anticonvulsant prophylaxis is rarely indicated. Parents should be advised to seek professional advice when the child develops fever so as to prevent the occurrence of high body temperatures.

A20   A

Viral croup, also known as acute laryngotracheobronchitis, is an age-specific viral syndrome characterised by acute laryngeal and subglottic swelling, resulting in hoarseness, cough, respiratory distress and inspiratory stridor. Mild croup does not require any specific drug treatment. If a child has croup that is severe or might cause complications, then the child can be given either oral prednisolone 1–2 mg/kg or oral dexamethasone 150 μg/kg as a single dose before transfer to hospital. When the condition is not effectively controlled with corticosteroid treatment, nebulised adrenaline (epinephrine) solution could be considered. The patient requires monitoring.

A21   C

Women suffering from diabetes mellitus or who are on lamotrigine (anti-epileptic agent) have an increased risk of conceiving a child with neural tube defects. Anti-epileptic agents, particularly carbamazepine, lamotrigine, oxcarbazepine, phenytoin and valproate, increase the risk of neural tube and other defects. To counteract the risk of neural tube defects, adequate folate supplements are advised for women before and during pregnancy, at a dose of 5 mg daily until week 12 of pregnancy.

A22   A

Exelon patches contain rivastigmine, which is indicated for mild-to-moderate Alzheimer's disease and in dementia associated with Parkinson's disease. When switching a patient from oral therapy to transdermal therapy, the 4.6 mg/24 hour patch is used for patients who are either taking 3–6 mg daily or who are taking 9 mg daily but are not tolerating the dose well. Patients who are taking 9 mg oral dose and who are tolerating the dose well or who are taking 12 mg daily are started on the 9.5 mg/24 hours patch. The patch is applied on the day after the last oral dose to clean, dry, non-hairy, non-irritated skin on the back, upper arm or chest. The patch should be changed after 24 hours. As with other transdermal drug-releasing patches, Exelon patches should be applied on a different area each time, avoiding the use of the same area for 14 days. Rivastigmine is a reversible, non-competitive inhibitor of acetylcholinesterases, and may cause gastrointestinal side-effects including gastric or duodenal ulceration as well as headache, drowsiness, tremor, asthenia, malaise, agitation, confusion, sweating and weight loss. Parameters that should be monitored include body weight.

A23   E

Rasilez contains aliskiren, which is a renin inhibitor used in hypertension as monotherapy or in combination with other antihypertensives. It is to be used with caution in patients taking concomitant diuretics, on a low-sodium diet or who are dehydrated and in patients with a glomerular filtration rate less than 30 mL/minute. Aliskiren may cause diarrhoea as a side-effect and it should be administered with or after food. It exists in two dosage strengths, 150 mg and 300 mg.

A24   C

Trabectedin is licensed for the treatment of advanced soft-tissue sarcoma when treatment with anthracyclines and ifosfamide has failed or is contraindicated. It is administered by intravenous infusion. Trabectedin may cause hepatobiliary disorders and for this reason hepatic function should be evaluated before starting treatment and during treatment. Dexamethasone is administered intravenously with trabectedin for its anti-emetic and hepatoprotective effects. As with other antineoplastic drugs, trabectedin causes nausea and vomiting and bone-marrow suppression as side-effects.

A25   E

Cerebral oedema is the excessive accumulation of fluid in the brain and is accompanied by an increase in intracranial pressure. It may be due to physical trauma, malignant disease, hypoxia at high altitude, poisoning, meningitis or stroke. Early treatment is essential and sometimes neurosurgical decompression or assisted ventilation may be necessary. Drug treatment consists of the administration of corticosteroids such as dexamethasone, particularlarly in oedema that is associated with malignant disease.

Intravenous administration of mannitol (osmotic diuretic) may be considered at a dose of 0.25–2 g/kg over 30–60 minutes.

A26   B

Obsessive compulsive disorder in an 8-year-old can be treated using fluvoxamine (selective serotonin reuptake inhibitor, SSRI). It is usually administered initially as 25 mg daily, and increased if necessary in steps of 25 mg every 4–7 days to a maximum of 200 mg daily. If there is no improvement within 10 weeks, treatment should be reconsidered. A selective serotonin reuptake inhibitor should not be started until 2 weeks after stopping a monoamine oxidase inhibitor (MAOI), and conversely a MAOI should not be started until at least a week after an SSRI has been stopped.

A27   B

Somatomedins are insulin-like polypeptide hormones that should be used with caution in diabetic patients since adjustment of antidiabetic therapy may be required. Before initiating therapy, a baseline ECG is recommended and, if abnormalities are identified, regular ECG monitoring during treatment is required. Somatomedins may cause tachycardia, cardiomegaly, ventricular hypertrophy and changes in blood glucose levels as side-effects.

A28   D

Erythropoeitins are used to treat symptomatic anaemia associated with erythropoietin deficiency in chronic renal failure and to shorten the period of symptomatic anaemia in patients receiving cytotoxic chemotherapy. It is not recommended for use in cancer patients who are not receiving chemotherapy. In cancer patients, the risk of thrombosis and related complications might be increased. The haemoglobin concentration should be maintained within the range of 10–12 g/100 mL – higher concentrations should be avoided to reduce risk of complications of therapy.

A29   B

Pegzerepoetin alfa (also known as methoxy polyethylene glycol-epoetin beta) is a continuous erythropoietin-receptor activator that is licensed for symptomatic anaemia associated with chronic kidney disease. It has a longer duration of action than epoetin and may be administered by subcutaneous or intravenous injection.

A30   A

Patients receiving oral anticoagulants such as warfarin may be liable to excessive bleeding after extraction of teeth or other dental surgery. For a patient who is on long-term warfarin, the INR should be assessed 72 hours before the dental procedure. This timeframe is recommended since it allows for sufficient time for dose modification if necessary. Patients undergoing minor dental procedures and dental extractions who have an INR below 4.0 do not require any dose adjustments. Drugs that have potentially serious interactions with warfarin include metronidazole, which is a commonly used anti-infective agent in dental practice because of its antiprotozoal activity. Metronidazole may enhance the effect of warfarin.

A31   A

Anaphylaxis is a severe allergic reaction that may follow drug administration or consumption of food items and insect stings. Adrenaline (epinephrine) is preferably given intramuscularly and dose is repeated according to blood pressure, pulse and respiratory function. Oxygen administration and intravenous fluids are also to be considered. An antihistamine, such as chlorphenamine given by slow intravenous or intramuscular injection is used as adjunctive treatment after adrenaline injections and continued for 1–2 days according to clinical response to prevent relapse.

A32   A

Rhabdomyolysis is the destruction of skeletal muscle tissues and may be associated with lipid-regulating drugs such as the fibrates and the statins. The risk of this side-effect is increased in patients with renal impairment and with hypothyroidism. Rhabdomyolysis may also occur with nicotinic acid, the antipsychotic aripiprazole, and the anaesthetic propofol.

A33   E

Tegretol consists of carbamazepine, which is an anti-epileptic drug. There is a clinically significant drug interaction between carbamazepine and clarithromycin (macrolide antibacterial agent) resulting in higher plasma concentrations of carbamazepine.

A34   B

Sofradex contains dexamethasone, framycetin and gramicidin and is indicated in otitis externa. Canesten contains clotrimazole and is indicated for fungal infections and may be used in otitis externa where a fungal infection is suspected. Nasonex contains mometasone, a corticosteroid, and is used in nasal allergy.

A35   B

There is an increased risk of hyperkalaemia when ciclosporin is given with Coversyl, which contains perindopril, an angiotensin-converting enzyme inhibitor. Risk of nephrotoxicity associated with ciclosporin is increased with concomitant use with quinolones. Ciproxin contains ciprofloxacin, which is a quinolone. Tenormin contains atenolol, which is a beta-adrenoceptor blocker and there are no interactions between these agents and ciclosporin.

A36   D

Malaria is a mosquito-borne disease caused by a parasite. The first symptoms of malaria tend to occur after the incubation period. The incubation period in most cases varies from 7 to 30 days. Symptoms include fever, chills and flu-like illness. Malaria is commonly encountered in Sub-Saharan and African regions.

A37   D

Travellers visiting remote, malarious areas for prolonged periods should carry standby treatment if they are likely to be more than 24 hours away from medical care. Patients should receive clear written instructions that urgent medical attention should be sought if fever (38°C or more) develops 7 days or more after arriving in a malarious area and that self-treatment is indicated if medical help is not available within 1 day of fever onset. A drug used for chemoprophylaxis should not be considered for standby medication.

A38   E

Mefloquine prophylaxis can be undertaken with caution in cardiac conduction disorders. It should be avoided in epilepsy, during pregnancy and breast-feeding and for 3 months after pregnancy.

A39   B

Pneumocystis carinii pneumonia occurs in immunocompromised patients and it hence is a common cause of pneumonia in AIDS. High doses of co-trimoxazole are indicated for treatment of mild-to-moderate pneumocystis pneumonia. This condition should be treated by those experienced in its management as it can be fatal.

A40   B

Pompholyx eczema is a special vesicular type of dermatitis affecting the hands and feet. It can be acute and persistent, characterised by many deep-seated, itchy, clear, tiny blisters. Later there may be scaling, fissures and thickening of the skin. Outbreaks usually last several weeks, and common sites include sides of the fingers, palms and, less often, on the soles. The aim of treatment is to prevent secondary infection and spontaneous resolution is expected within 2 or 3 weeks. If, however, it persists, it may be necessary to use short courses of corticosteroid creams. It is an inflammatory reaction and there is no underlying infective component.

A41   A

Arnica has been used for medicinal purposes. It can be applied topically as a cream, ointment, liniment, salve or tincture, to soothe muscle aches, reduce inflammation and heal wounds. It is often used for injuries such as sprains and bruises. Arnica is primarily restricted to topical (external) use because it can cause serious side-effects when ingested. Arnica consists of a number of flavonoid glycosides and terpenoids.

A42   A

Anogenital warts (condylomata acuminata) are caused by the human papillomavirus and are usually sexually transmitted. The average incubation period is 2–3 months. During pregnancy, the warts may become more widespread, favouring an even more rapid growth. Spontaneous resolution may occur. However, they tend to recur in some patients.

A43   C

Imiquimod cream is used for the treatment of external anogenital warts, where it may be used for both keratinised and non-keratinised lesions. It is also used in superficial basal cell carcinoma and actinic keratosis. Side-effects include local reactions such as itching, burning sensation, erythema, erosion, oedema, excoriation and stabbing and, less commonly, local ulceration. Patients should be advised to rub it in and to allow it to stay on the treated area for 6–10 hours for warts. The cream should then be washed off with mild soap and water.

A44   A

Silver nitrate, which is a caustic agent, is available as a stick or pen in combination with potassium nitrate and is suitable for the removal of warts on the hands and feet. It should be used with caution and patients are advised to protect the surrounding skin, as it can cause chemical burns. It can also cause staining of skin and fabric.

A45   B

Tetracosactide (tetracosactrin) is an analogue of corticotrophin (ACTH) and is used to test adrenocortical function. It is administered by intramuscular injection. Side-effects are very similar to those with corticosteroids.

A46 C

Huntington's chorea is a rare, dominantly inherited, progressive disease characterised by chorea (brief involuntary jerky muscle contractions) and dementia. It has an insidious onset and usually occurs between 30 and 50 years of age. Symptoms include uncontrolled movements, personality disorders, severe depression and anxiety.

A47 C

In Huntington's chorea, tetrabenazine is used to control movement disorders. It probably causes a depletion of nerve endings of dopamine. However, it has a useful action in only a proportion of patients and its use may be limited by the development of depression, a symptom that may already be present due to the underlying disease itself.

A48 D

Whipple's disease is a rare malabsorption syndrome, which usually occurs in men aged 30–60 years of age. It is caused by a bacterium, *Tropheryma whippelii*, which infiltrates the mucosa of the small intestine. The symptoms are characterised by arthritis, steatorrhea, weight loss, abdominal pain, fever and weakness. Treatment consists of prolonged administration of antibacterial drugs and the correction of nutritional deficiencies.

A49 C

Gelatin is a plasma substitute. Plasma substitutes should not be used to maintain plasma volume in burns or peritonitis. In these scenarios albumin should be given. Close monitoring, including monitoring of fluid and electrolyte balance and urine output, is required in patients being administered plasma and plasma substitutes. Plasma substitutes should also be used with caution in patients with cardiac disease, liver disease or renal impairment.

A50 A

Midazolam is a water-soluble benzodiazepine that is often used in preference to diazepam, since recovery is faster than with diazepam. It is indicated for the induction of anaesthesia, and in sedation with amnesia or in intensive care.

A51 D

Infliximab is licensed for the management of severe active Crohn's disease and in rheumatoid arthritis. Maintenance therapy with infliximab should be considered for patients who respond to the initial induction course. Infliximab is administered by intravenous infusion and, for severe active Crohn's disease, it is started initially with 5 mg/kg and then 5 mg/kg 2 weeks after the initial dose.

A52 B

Glyceryl trinitrate can be used topically in the treatment of anal fissures. Being a nitrovasodilator when applied topically, glyceryl trinitrate tends to cause relaxation of the anal sphincter. It is applied to the anal canal until the pain stops.

A53 B

Omalizumab is a monoclonal antibody that binds to immunoglobulin E. It is used as additional therapy in asthma patients who have a proven IgE-mediated sensitivity to inhaled allergens and who are presenting with severe, persistent, uncontrolled asthma. It is administered by subcutaneous injection and the dose is calculated based on the immunoglobulin E concentration and body weight.

A54 C

Abciximab is a monoclonal antibody that binds to glycoprotein IIb/IIIa receptors, thereby blocking the binding of fibrinogen to receptors on platelets. It acts as by preventing platelet aggregation. It is used as an adjunct to heparin and aspirin in high-risk patients undergoing percutaneous transluminal coronary intervention. Baseline prothrombin time, activated clotting time, activated partial thromboplastin time, platelet count, haemoglobin and haematocrit should be measured at baseline. Patient monitoring is required after the start of treatment.

A55   D

Avandia contains rosiglitazone, which is a thiazolidinedione that is used as oral antidiabetic therapy. Thiazolidinediones reduce peripheral insulin resistance, resulting in reductions in blood-glucose concentrations. Inadequate response to oral antidiabetic therapy indicates failing insulin release and the impact of the introduction of rosiglitazone is of limited benefit on patient outcomes. Insulin should be considered.

A56   D

Avandia (rosiglitazone) as with other thiazolidinediones is used either as monotherapy or in combination with either metformin or a sulphonylurea. A disadvantage of rosiglitazone is the risk of heart failure as a side-effect. This risk is increased when rosiglitazone is used in patients with cardiovascular disease and when used in combination with insulin. Blood-glucose control may deteriorate temporarily when a thiazolidinedione is substituted for an oral antidiabetic agent.

A57   E

Dexamethasone is a fluorinated potent corticosteroid that readily crosses the placenta in pregnancy. Prednisolone is preferred during pregnancy since 88% is inactivated as it crosses the placenta.

A58   C

Bupropion should not be administered with sedating antihistamines because of the increased risk of seizures. Bupropion is used for smoking cessation therapy and may cause insomnia as a side-effect. Patients are advised to avoid taking bupropion dose at bedtime.

A59   D

Varenicline is a selective nicotine receptor partial agonist that is used in smoking cessation. It is started 1–2 weeks before target stop date. It may cause gastrointestinal disturbances, dry mouth, taste disturbance and, less commonly, aphthous stomatitis.

A60 E

Tibolone is a product that has oestrogenic, progestogenic and weak androgenic activity that is used for the short-term treatment of symptoms of oestrogen deficiency. Tibolone should not be used in premenopausal women since it may cause irregular vaginal bleeding in the initial stages of treatment, which in these patients may be difficult to identify. Hormone replacement therapy is associated with an increased risk of venous thromboembolism. The limited data available do not suggest an increased risk of thromboembolism with tibolone, when compared with combined HRT, or in women not taking hormone replacement therapy.

A61 B

Bonviva consists of ibandronic acid, a bisphosphonate and is available as 150 mg tablets and 1 mg/mL injection. Patients receiving the oral formulation for the treatment of postmenopausal osteoporosis are advised to take one tablet once a month. Absorption of bisphosphonates from the gastrointestinal tract may be effected by food or other administered drugs. Therefore patients are advised to take the Bonviva 150 mg tablet at least 1 hour before breakfast or another oral medicine and to continue standing or sitting upright for at least 1 hour after administration.

A62 A

Actonel contains risedronate sodium, a bisphosphonate. Osteonecrosis of the jaw has been reported in patients receiving oral bisphosphonates. Adequate oral hygiene should be maintained during and after treatment with bisphosphonates, including Actonel. Preventive dental treatment should be considered before starting bisphosphonates. Patient should be advised to maintain adequate oral hygiene during treatment.

A63 B

Bevacizumab is a monoclonal antibody that inhibits vascular endothelial growth factor. It should be used with caution in patients with a history of hypertension because of an increased risk of proteinuria and in patients with uncontrolled hypertension. Side-effects that may be expected include hypertension and congestive heart failure. One of the parameters that should be monitored during treatment is blood pressure.

A64   B

When azathioprine is administered concomitantly with allopurinol, there is a risk of enhanced effects and increased toxicity of azathioprine. Doses of azathioprine should be reduced to one quarter of the usual dose. Both allopurinol and azathioprine may cause hypersensitivity reactions.

A65   A

Daunorubicin is an anthracycline antibiotic used in chemotherapy. It is diluted with infusion fluid to a concentration of 1 mg/mL and given over 20 minutes to reduce the occurrence of irritation. A liposomal formulation is also available.

A66   A

Methotrexate is an antimetabolite drug that is excreted primarily by the kidney. It is contraindicated in significant renal impairment and in hepatic impairment. It is nephrotoxic and accumulation may occur in renal impairment. Dose should be reduced in renal impairment that is not severe and drug should be avoided if creatinine clearance is less than 20 mL/minute.

A67   C

Habitual abortion is repeated spontaneous abortion. Suturing of the cervix may prevent abortion in cases of cervical incompetence. Administration of low-dose aspirin and a prophylactic dose of a low-molecular-weight heparin may be beneficial in pregnant women having antiphospholipid syndrome and who have suffered recurrent miscarriage, since aspirin and heparin decrease the risk of fetal loss. Dydrogesterone is a progestogen analogue that, although it has been used for the prevention of spontaneous abortion in women with a history of recurrent miscarriage, is not recommended for use in this scenario, because of lack of evidence.

A68 A

Severe pain in the loin lasting several hours and which is recurring requires referral to investigate underlying cause. One of the systems that need to be investigated is the renal system. Pain originating from kidney disorders and renal colic (renal calculi) initially presents with loin pain and may radiate to the back or spread downwards to the iliac fossa, suprapubic area and in males into the scrotum.

A69 A

Trimipramine is a tricyclic antidepressant with sedative properties that is used in the management of depression. As with other tricyclic antidepressants, trimipramine has antimuscarinic activity and therefore side-effects include dry mouth, blurred vision, constipation and urinary retention.

A70 B

Lithium is used in the prophylaxis and treatment of mania and in the prophylaxis of bipolar disorders and recurrent depression. Lithium should be stopped 24 hours before major surgery but the normal dose can be continued for minor surgery, with careful monitoring of fluids and electrolytes. After major surgery, renal function is reduced and this may compromise clearance of lithium. Lithium is a drug with a narrow therapeutic index and it should be avoided if possible in patients with renal impairment. Renal function should be tested before initiating treatment. If lithium is given to patients with renal impairment, a reduced dose should be used and serum lithium concentrations should be monitored closely.

A71 A

Lithium should be used with caution in conditions with sodium imbalance, such as Addison's disease.

A72 B

Nitrous oxide is used for the maintenance of anaesthesia as part of a combination of drugs because, owing to its lack of potency, it cannot be used as a sole anaesthetic. Using nitrous oxide at a concentration of 50–66% in oxygen, a reduced dose of other anaesthetics can be adopted.

A73   D

Desflurane is a rapid-acting, volatile, liquid anaesthetic. However, compared with isoflurane, it has a lower potency. Desflurane is not used for the induction of anaesthesia, as it is irritant to the upper respiratory tract leading to cough, apnoea, laryngospasm and increased secretions.

A74   D

Prilocaine is a local anaesthetic of low toxicity, which should be avoided in severe or untreated hypertension, severe heart disease and in patients using drugs that may cause methaemoglobinaemia. Prilocaine may cause ocular toxicity, which has been reported with the use of the product in excessively high doses during ophthalmic procedures.

A75   A

Cocaine readily penetrates mucous membranes and is an effective topical local anaesthetic that demonstrates intensive vasoconstrictor action. It has stimulant effects on the central nervous system and is a drug of addiction. It causes agitation, dilated pupils, tachycardia, hypertension, hallucinations, hyperthermia, hypertonia, hyperreflexia and cardiac effects.

A76   C

Lantus contains insulin glargine, which is a human insulin analogue that provides a prolonged duration of action and requires once daily administration. It is recommended for patients who are suffering from recurrent symptomatic hypoglycaemia. Because of the once-daily dosage regimen it is useful in patients who have difficulty with handling insulin administration. Some patients may be administered a combination of insulin therapy and oral antidiabetics including metformin (biguanide).

A77   B

Giant cell arteritis (cranial or temporal arteritis) is an inflammatory condition that may affect any of the large arteries, especially the temporal and occipital arteries. The thickened temporal arteries may be tender and non-pulsatile, with erythema and oedema of the overlying skin. Early treatment with high-dose corticosteroids such as prednisolone is essential and should be continued for a minimum of 2–3 years at a reduced dose.

A78   D

Flecainide is a drug used for arrhythmias and is of particular use in ventricular arrhythmias and paroxysmal atrial fibrillation. Flecainide has a membrane-stabilising activity. Use of flecainide may precipitate serious arrhythmias, even in patients with no history of cardiovascular disease and with otherwise normal hearts.

A79   D

Amiodarone is a drug used for arrhythmias, which has very similar properties to flecainide. Both drugs may cause pneumonitis as a side-effect but risk is lower with flecainide. Signs of pneumonitis include progressive shortness of breath or cough.

A80   B

Disulfiram is used as an adjunct in the management of alcohol dependence. It is contraindicated in patients with a history of cerebrovascular accident, cardiac failure, coronary artery disease, hypertension and psychosis. Side-effects that may be present include initial drowsiness and fatigue, nausea, vomiting, halitosis, reduced libido, psychotic reactions, allergic dermatitis, peripheral neuritis and hepatic cell damage.

A81–85

Onychomycosis is a fungal nail infection. In severe cases, oral antifungals are recommended as first-line agents. Oral triazole antifungals such as itraconazole (Sporanox capsules) as well as terbinafine (Lamisil tablets) are recommended. Treatment with itraconazole poses a lesser burden to patients in terms of number of doses required when compared with terbinafine. When used topically, imidazole antifungal agents such as miconazole (Daktarin cream) and ketoconazole (Nizoral cream) are less effective in severe onychomycosis and twice-daily administration is required at least. Aciclovir (Zovirax cream) is an antiviral agent and does not provide any clinical input in onychomycosis.

A81   3

A82   2

A83   4

A84   1

A85   5

A86–89

Mirtazapine is indicated for major depression. Its side-effects include sedation and, less commonly, dizziness, abnormal dreams (rarely) and, very rarely, angle-closure glaucoma.

A86   3

A87   4

A88   2

A89   1

A90–92

In patients allergic to penicillin, macrolides are usually indicated in mild respiratory tract infections. Zithromax contains azithromycin, which is a macrolide that may be indicated for respiratory tract infections. As opposed to clarithromycin (another macrolide), azithromycin does not present any significant clinical interaction with phenytoin. Ciproxin contains ciprofloxacin, which is a quinolone. When ciprofloxacin is used in patients who are taking phenytoin, the plasma concentration of phenytoin may be increased or decreased. In addition, quinolones should be used with caution in patients with a history of epilepsy, since they lower the seizure threshold. Flagyl, which contains metronidazole, is not normally used in respiratory tract infections, since metronidazole is particulary active against anaerobic bacteria and protozoa. Concomitant use of metronidazole and phenytoin is associated with a significant clinical interaction, resulting in inhibition of metabolism of phenytoin.

A90 2

A91 3

A92 1

A93–97

Cefalexin is a first-generation cephalosporin and therefore an alternative preparation would be Zinnat tablets, which contains cefuroxime, a second-generation cephalosporin. A penicillin such as Augmentin, which contains co-amoxiclav, can be an appropriate alternative since it provides a very similar spectrum of activity. Klaricid contains clarithromycin, which is a macrolide. Utinor contains norfloxacin, which is a quinolone that is effective in uncomplicated urinary-tract infections. Rocephin contains ceftriaxone, which is a third-generation cephalosporin that is available for parenteral administration only.

A93 2

A94 3

A95 5

A96 4

A97 1

A98–100

In mild-to-moderate acne topical treatment such as benzoyl peroxide (Panoxyl gel) is usually recommended, followed by clindamycin (Dalacin capsules). Roaccutane capsules, which contain isotretinoin, are reserved for more severe cases of acne.

A98   2

A99   1

A100 3

Section 2

Closed-book Questions

Test 5

Questions

Questions 1–38

Directions: Each of the questions or incomplete statements is followed by five suggested answers. Select the best answer in each case.

Q1   Which one of the following is the most appropriate for the management of an upper respiratory tract infection in a patient who is allergic to penicillin?

A   ❑ sodium fusidate
B   ❑ trimethoprim
C   ❑ clarithromycin
D   ❑ cefuroxime
E   ❑ co-amoxiclav

Q2   The cautionary label 'May cause drowsiness' should be used in all of the following EXCEPT:

A   ❑ codeine
B   ❑ sumatriptan
C   ❑ tramadol
D   ❑ fentanyl
E   ❑ diclofenac

Q3   The usual expiration date that should be placed on a cream prepared in a pharmacy is:

A   ❑ 1 week
B   ❑ 2 weeks
C   ❑ 4 weeks
D   ❑ 8 weeks
E   ❑ 12 weeks

Q4   A 61-year-old retired person receiving 20 mg fluvastatin daily may report:

   A   ❑ myalgia
   B   ❑ drowsiness
   C   ❑ palpitations
   D   ❑ constipation
   E   ❑ pruritus

Q5   Which of the following is particularly useful in a hypoglycaemic reaction?

   A   ❑ sparkling water
   B   ❑ still water
   C   ❑ sweets
   D   ❑ bread
   E   ❑ salad

Q6   A pharmacist prepares a saline solution by adding 1 g of sodium chloride in 100 mL water. What is the percentage of sodium chloride present?

   A   ❑ 10%
   B   ❑ 1%
   C   ❑ 0.1%
   D   ❑ 0.01%
   E   ❑ 100%

Q7   Thiazide diuretics should usually be avoided in patients with:

   A   ❑ hypertension
   B   ❑ hypernatraemia
   C   ❑ hypercalcaemia
   D   ❑ oedema
   E   ❑ heart failure

Q8   Alcoholic drink should be avoided with:

A   ❏ amoxicillin
B   ❏ metronidazole
C   ❏ ciprofloxacin
D   ❏ doxycycline
E   ❏ co-trimoxazole

Q9   Which of these components should NOT be included in a preparation during pregnancy?

A   ❏ zinc
B   ❏ iron
C   ❏ folic acid
D   ❏ vitamin A
E   ❏ vitamin E

Q10   A patient is prescribed itraconazole. Which drug may interact with itraconazole?

A   ❏ paracetamol
B   ❏ ibuprofen
C   ❏ digoxin
D   ❏ co-amoxiclav
E   ❏ enalapril

Q11   How many tablets of prednisolone 5 mg should be dispensed to a patient who has been prescribed prednisolone 25 mg for 5 days:

A   ❏ 25
B   ❏ 125
C   ❏ 5
D   ❏ 50
E   ❏ 45

Q12   All of the following are oral antidiabetic drugs classified as sulphony-lureas EXCEPT:

     A   ❑ glibenclamide
     B   ❑ glimepiride
     C   ❑ gliclazide
     D   ❑ tolbutamide
     E   ❑ metformin

Q13   A patient is prescribed 1 L dextrose 5% with potassium chloride over 6 hours. Treatment is started at 8.00 am. At noon the patient is changed to 1 L normal saline over 12 hours. The patient's total intra-venous fluid intake in the period 8.00 am to midnight is:

     A   ❑ 666 mL
     B   ❑ 1000 mL
     C   ❑ 1666 mL
     D   ❑ 2000 mL
     E   ❑ 2500 mL

Q14   Which preparation could be used systemically in the treatment of acne?

     A   ❑ azelaic acid
     B   ❑ clindamycin
     C   ❑ salicylic acid
     D   ❑ benzoyl peroxide
     E   ❑ triclosan

Q15   Which of the following active ingredients is NOT used for the man-agement of cough?

     A   ❑ codeine
     B   ❑ dextromethorphan
     C   ❑ pholcodine
     D   ❑ vitamin C
     E   ❑ diphenhydramine

Q16   Amitriptyline is classified as a (an):

A   ❑ atypical antidepressant
B   ❑ tricyclic antidepressant
C   ❑ antipsychotic drug
D   ❑ antimanic drug
E   ❑ hypnotic

Q17   A patient has been prescribed naproxen 0.25 g b.d. for 7 days. Naproxen 500 mg scored tablets are available. How many tablets should be dispensed?

A   ❑ 14
B   ❑ 12
C   ❑ 10
D   ❑ 7
E   ❑ 4

Q18   The dose of diazepam for children in febrile convulsions is 250 μg/kg. What is the appropriate dose for a child weighing 25 kg?

A   ❑ 6250 mg
B   ❑ 6.25 mg
C   ❑ 62.5 mg
D   ❑ 10 mg
E   ❑ 625 mg

Q19   Tapeworm infections are caused by:

A   ❑ *Taenia solium*
B   ❑ tinea pedis
C   ❑ *Yersinia pestis*
D   ❑ *Candida albicans*
E   ❑ *Chlamydia trachomitis*

Q20   A patient weighs 85 kg and is 1.74 m tall. The patient's body mass index is:

A   ❏   0.02
B   ❏   0.04
C   ❏   2.8
D   ❏   28
E   ❏   48

Q21   Which of the following conditions could NOT be caused by a bacterial infection?

A   ❏   septicaemia
B   ❏   scabies
C   ❏   endocarditis
D   ❏   peritonitis
E   ❏   shigellosis

Q22   Salbutamol:

A   ❏   is a selective beta$_2$-adrenoceptor stimulant
B   ❏   has a long duration of action
C   ❏   should not be used in conjunction with beclometasone
D   ❏   may cause drowsiness
E   ❏   may precipitate oral candidiasis

Q23   Characteristic symptoms of hyperglycaemia include all EXCEPT:

A   ❏   weakness
B   ❏   thirst
C   ❏   visual disturbances
D   ❏   ketonuria
E   ❏   dysuria

Q24 Ergotamine:

A   ❏ may cause tingling of extremities
B   ❏ is used in the prophylaxis of migraine
C   ❏ has anti-emetic properties
D   ❏ may be used in hepatic impairment
E   ❏ is a 5HT$_1$ agonist

Q25 Drugs used in the treatment of parkinsonism include all EXCEPT:

A   ❏ co-careldopa
B   ❏ amantadine
C   ❏ entacapone
D   ❏ bromocriptine
E   ❏ chlorpromazine

Q26 Oxytocin is used in:

A   ❏ labour induction
B   ❏ premature labour
C   ❏ ductus arteriosus
D   ❏ vaginal atrophy
E   ❏ urinary retention

Q27 Which of the following drugs is NOT liable to cause dry mouth?

A   ❏ trihexyphenidyl
B   ❏ cinnarizine
C   ❏ imipramine
D   ❏ sumatriptan
E   ❏ orphenadrine

Q28   A patient is administered 500 mL normal saline over 4 hours using 10
drops/mL infusion set. The infusion rate in drops/minute is:

A   ❏ 2
B   ❏ 5
C   ❏ 10
D   ❏ 13
E   ❏ 21

Q29   Which of the following is of value in the management of furuncles?

A   ❏ hydrocortisone
B   ❏ fusidic acid
C   ❏ aciclovir
D   ❏ promethazine
E   ❏ zinc oxide

Q30   Which one of the following drugs is NOT likely to cause sensitisation?

A   ❏ mepyramine
B   ❏ prilocaine
C   ❏ benzocaine
D   ❏ lidocaine
E   ❏ hydrocortisone

Q31   A mother comes to the pharmacy with her 3-year-old son who suffers
from allergic rhinitis. Which of the following is an appropriate product to be recommended to counteract the rhinorrhoea?

A   ❏ benzydamine spray
B   ❏ budesonide nasal spray
C   ❏ mupirocin nasal ointment
D   ❏ sodium chloride spray
E   ❏ xylometazoline nasal drops

Q32   Constituents of oral rehydration salts include all EXCEPT:

A   ❑ sodium chloride
B   ❑ glucose
C   ❑ potassium chloride
D   ❑ sodium citrate
E   ❑ magnesium hydroxide

Q33   In cough, which of the following constituents is used to reduce sputum viscosity:

A   ❑ promethazine
B   ❑ pholcodine
C   ❑ dextromethorphan
D   ❑ carbocisteine
E   ❑ chlorphenamine

Q34   For which of the following drugs is a long-acting oral formulation available:

A   ❑ prednisolone
B   ❑ domperidone
C   ❑ diclofenac
D   ❑ paracetamol
E   ❑ gentamicin

Q35   Common side-effects of bumetanide include all EXCEPT:

A   ❑ hypokalaemia
B   ❑ hyponatraemia
C   ❑ gynaecomastia
D   ❑ gout
E   ❑ hypotension

Q36   Baclofen is a (an):

A   ❏ prostaglandin
B   ❏ corticosteroid
C   ❏ skeletal muscle relaxant
D   ❏ non-steroidal anti-inflammatory drug
E   ❏ opioid analgesic

Q37   Topical products used in hyperhidrosis may contain aluminium chloride as a (an):

A   ❏ desloughing agent
B   ❏ antiperspirant
C   ❏ astringent
D   ❏ antifungal
E   ❏ barrier preparation

Q38   Agents that could be recommended for otitis externa include all EXCEPT:

A   ❏ hydrocortisone
B   ❏ docusate sodium
C   ❏ gentamicin
D   ❏ neomycin
E   ❏ clioquinol

Questions 39–51

Directions: Each group of questions below consists of five lettered headings followed by a list of numbered questions. For each numbered question select the one heading that is most closely related to it. Each heading may be used once, more than once, or not at all.

Questions 39–41 concern the following conditions:

A   ❑ Hyperkeratosis
B   ❑ Ascites
C   ❑ Peripheral neuropathy
D   ❑ Nocturia
E   ❑ Paget's disease

Select, from A to E, which one of the above:

Q39   may be present in hepatic failure

Q40   is a complication of rheumatoid arthritis

Q41   may predispose to secondary osteoarthritis

Questions 42–44 concern the following abbreviations:

A   ❑ NIDDM
B   ❑ COPD
C   ❑ PMH
D   ❑ PND
E   ❑ CAPD

Select, from A to E, the abbreviation corresponding to the descriptions below:

Q42   past medical history

Q43   non-insulin dependent diabetes mellitus

Q44   continuous ambulatory peritoneal dialysis

Questions 45–48 concern the following drugs:

A   ❑ ampicillin
B   ❑ atazanavir
C   ❑ nystatin
D   ❑ choline salicylate
E   ❑ chlorhexidine

Select, from A to E, which one of the above:

Q45   provides analgesic action

Q46   may be used in the treatment of intestinal candidiasis

Q47   inhibits plaque formation on teeth

Q48   may cause brown staining of teeth

Questions 49–51 concern the following drugs:

A   ❑ prednisolone
B   ❑ triamcinolone
C   ❑ hydrocortisone butyrate
D   ❑ hydrocortisone
E   ❑ fluticasone

Select, from A to E, which one of the above:

Q49   is administered by inhalation

Q50   is commonly used orally for long-term disease suppression

Q51   is available as a low-potency corticosteroid for topical administration to the skin

Questions 52–79

Directions: For each of the questions below, ONE or MORE of the responses is (are) correct. Decide which of the responses is (are) correct. Then choose:

A   ❏ if 1, 2 and 3 are correct
B   ❏ if 1 and 2 only are correct
C   ❏ if 2 and 3 only are correct
D   ❏ if 1 only is correct
E   ❏ if 3 only is correct

Directions summarised				
A	**B**	**C**	**D**	**E**
1, 2, 3	1, 2 only	2, 3 only	1 only	3 only

Q52 Which of the following is (are) recognised treatments for prolonged febrile convulsions?

1   ❏ diazepam
2   ❏ levodopa
3   ❏ phenytoin

Q53 Clinical features of glaucoma include:

1   ❏ ocular pain
2   ❏ visual disturbances
3   ❏ mucous discharge

Q54 Predisposing factors for low back pain include:

1   ❏ trauma
2   ❏ osteoporosis
3   ❏ angina

Q55 Side-effects of loperamide include:

1 ❏ diarrhoea
2 ❏ skin reactions
3 ❏ abdominal cramps

Q56 Sympathomimetics include:

1 ❏ dobutamine
2 ❏ isoprenaline
3 ❏ orphenadrine

Q57 Drugs used in the prophylaxis of angina include:

1 ❏ atenolol
2 ❏ isosorbide dinitrate
3 ❏ digoxin

Q58 Therapeutic uses of angiotensin-converting enzyme inhibitors include:

1 ❏ hypertension
2 ❏ heart failure
3 ❏ arrhythmias

Q59 Treatment of gout includes:

1 ❏ indapamide
2 ❏ allopurinol
3 ❏ naproxen

Q60 Gentamicin:

1 ❏ is active against some Gram-positive organisms
2 ❏ is active against anaerobic bacteria
3 ❏ is a cephalosporin

Q61   A patient information leaflet:

1   ❑ is addressed to the prescriber
2   ❑ is only available for medicines presented in bulk dispensing packs
3   ❑ usually includes the recommended International Non-proprietary Name (rINN) of the drug

Q62   Tinnitus:

1   ❑ is the perception of sound in the ears
2   ❑ may be caused by aspirin overdosage
3   ❑ indicates an inflammatory process in the ear

Q63   Common signs of adverse drug reactions include:

1   ❑ urticaria
2   ❑ fever
3   ❑ maculopapular eruptions

Q64   Advantages of selective serotonin re-uptake inhibitors over the tricyclic antidepressants include:

1   ❑ fewer antimuscarinic side-effects
2   ❑ less cardiotoxicity in overdosage
3   ❑ being more effective

Q65   Risk factors for the development of pressure ulcers may include:

1   ❑ immobility
2   ❑ incontinence
3   ❑ cough

Q66   Clinical trials:

1   ❑ assess safety and efficacy of a drug in humans
2   ❑ involve different phases
3   ❑ follow good clinical practice standards

Q67   Iron salts:

1   ❑ should be given by mouth unless there are good reasons for using another route
2   ❑ in the form of ferric salts are better absorbed than the ferrous salts
3   ❑ should always be taken on an empty stomach

Q68   Which of the following drug(s) is (are) likely to be prescribed in amen-orrhoea?

1   ❑ dydrogesterone
2   ❑ non-steroidal anti-inflammatory drugs
3   ❑ iron supplements

Q69   Disadvantages of depot parenteral preparations include:

1   ❑ increased frequency of dosing compared with oral route
2   ❑ being less effective than other presentations
3   ❑ administration that may not be acceptable to the patient

Q70   Cetirizine:

1   ❑ is a non-sedating antihistamine
2   ❑ is indicated in symptomatic relief of hay fever
3   ❑ is an active metabolite of fexofenadine

Q71   Rubefacients:

1   ❑ act by counter-irritation
2   ❑ should be avoided on broken skin
3   ❑ are exemplified by ketoprofen

Q72   Thyroxine:

1   ❑ is indicated in hyperthyroidism
2   ❑ treatment should not exceed 1 week
3   ❑ should preferably be taken in the morning

Q73 Emollients:

1 ❏ provide a long duration of action
2 ❏ may be applied up to twice daily
3 ❏ are useful in eczema

Q74 Which preparation(s) is (are) available for scalp application?

1 ❏ ketoconazole
2 ❏ coal tar
3 ❏ amoxicillin

Q75 Patients presenting with diarrhoea should be referred if it:

1 ❏ persists for more than 24 hours in infants under 1 year
2 ❏ occurs in babies under 3 months
3 ❏ is associated with vomiting

Q76 Preparations that could be recommended to a patient who has athlete's foot include:

1 ❏ salicylic acid
2 ❏ tolnaftate
3 ❏ clotrimazole

Q77 Viral meningitis:

1 ❏ is an infection of brain and spinal cord parenchyma
2 ❏ is not always associated with high fever
3 ❏ is associated with the occurrence of headache

Q78 Which of the following drugs would be effective as a bowel cleanser prior to colonoscopy?

1 ❏ magnesium salts
2 ❏ glycerin
3 ❏ ispaghula husk

Q79 Cough may be associated with:

1 ❏ respiratory infections
2 ❏ lung cancer
3 ❏ smoking

Questions 80–84

Directions: The following questions consist of a first statement followed by a second statement. Decide whether the first statement is true or false. Decide whether the second statement is true or false. Then choose:

A   ❏ if both statements are true and the second statement is a *correct explanation* of the first statement
B   ❏ if both statements are true but the second statement *is NOT a correct explanation* of the first statement
C   ❏ if the first statement is true but the second statement is false
D   ❏ if the first statement is false but the second statement is true
E   ❏ if both statements are false

Directions summarised			
	First statement	**Second statement**	
A	True	True	Second statement is a *correct explanation* of the first
B	True	True	Second statement is *NOT a correct explanation* of the first
C	True	False	
D	False	True	
E	False	False	

Q80   During pregnancy, diet should consist of foods rich in starch, vitamins and minerals. During pregnancy, food containing sugars, fats and refined carbohydrates should be limited.

Q81   Soft-textured toothbrushes are more efficient in removing plaque than medium-textured brushes. Hard-textured brushes may cause gingival trauma.

Q82   Exercise is contraindicated in controlled angina. Swimming is greatly associated with exercise-induced asthma.

Q83   Support bandages provide support to an injured area during movement. Support bandages reduce risk of infection.

Q84   Calamine lotion may be applied after a jellyfish sting. Jellyfish release histamine that causes erythema.

Questions 85–100

Directions: These questions involve cases. Read the prescription or case and answer the questions.

Questions 85–89: Use the prescription below

Patient's name: . . . .

Age: 5 years
Paracetamol 250 mg suppositories
q.d.s.   m. 20
Co-amoxiclav 457 mg/5 mL suspension
5 mL b.d.   m. 1 bottle

Doctor's signature: . . . .

Q85   Co-amoxiclav is a combination of clavulanic acid and

A   ❑ amoxicillin
B   ❑ ampicillin
C   ❑ cefuroxime
D   ❑ flucloxacillin
E   ❑ pivampicillin

Q86   Co-amoxiclav suspension:

1   ❑ should be reconstituted before dispensing
2   ❑ should be agitated before use
3   ❑ should be administered twice daily

A   ❑ 1, 2, 3
B   ❑ 1, 2 only
C   ❑ 2, 3 only
D   ❑ 1 only
E   ❑ 3 only

Q87   For this patient, dose by rectum of paracetamol suppositories is:

A   ❑ 125–250 mg up to four times daily
B   ❑ 250–500 mg up to four times daily
C   ❑ 125–250 mg up to six times daily
D   ❑ 60–100 mg up to four times daily
E   ❑ up to 4000 mg per day

Q88   Parent may be advised to:

1   ❑ monitor body temperature
2   ❑ keep child well hydrated
3   ❑ discontinue use of co-amoxiclav suspension as soon as symptoms subside

A   ❑ 1, 2, 3
B   ❑ 1, 2 only
C   ❑ 2, 3 only
D   ❑ 1 only
E   ❑ 3 only

Q89   Paracetamol suppositories may have been preferred to oral suspension because:

1   ❑ there is vomiting
2   ❑ child is reluctant to take medication
3   ❑ there is diarrhoea

A   ❑ 1, 2, 3
B   ❑ 1, 2 only
C   ❑ 2, 3 only
D   ❑ 1 only
E   ❑ 3 only

Questions 90–92:

A patient presents with symptoms of cystitis. The prescriber recommends an antibacterial drug.

For the following drugs, place your order of preference assigning 1 to the product that should be recommended as first choice and 3 to the product that should be recommended as a last choice.

Q90   amoxicillin

Q91   doxycycline

Q92   itraconazole

Questions 93–94: Use the patient profile below

Patient medication profile

Patient's name: . . . .

Age: 72 years
Medical history: venous thrombosis
Medication record: warfarin 7.5 mg daily

The patient comes to the pharmacy complaining of sore throat, fever and rhinorrhoea.

Q93   What lines of actions would you follow?

1   ❑ dispense paracetamol
2   ❑ dispense a topical nasal decongestant
3   ❑ alter dose of warfarin

A   ❑ 1, 2, 3
B   ❑ 1, 2 only
C   ❑ 2, 3 only
D   ❑ 1 only
E   ❑ 3 only

Q94   What advice should be given?

1   ❑ seek advice from a general practitioner immediately
2   ❑ monitor INR daily
3   ❑ seek advice if condition gets worse

A   ❑ 1, 2, 3
B   ❑ 1, 2 only
C   ❑ 2, 3 only
D   ❑ 1 only
E   ❑ 3 only

Questions 95–100: Use the prescription below

Patient's name: . . . .

Chloramphenicol eye drops
b.d.   m. 1 bottle
Chloramphenicol eye ointment
nocte   m. 1 pack

Doctor's signature: . . . .

Q95   Conjunctivitis is inflammation of the:

A   ❑ eyelid margins
B   ❑ conjunctiva
C   ❑ iris
D   ❑ lacrymal sac
E   ❑ meibomian glands

Q96   Chloramphenicol:

1   ❑ has a broad spectrum
2   ❑ should not be used in superficial eye infections
3   ❑ should not be used in undiagnosed 'red eye'

A   ❑ 1, 2, 3
B   ❑ 1, 2 only
C   ❑ 2, 3 only
D   ❑ 1 only
E   ❑ 3 only

Q97   Common side-effects experienced with chloramphenicol eye preparations may include:

1   ❏ transient stinging
2   ❏ agranulocytosis
3   ❏ photophobia

A   ❏ 1, 2, 3
B   ❏ 1, 2 only
C   ❏ 2, 3 only
D   ❏ 1 only
E   ❏ 3 only

Q98   Patient should be advised to:

1   ❏ apply drops morning and midday
2   ❏ apply ointment at night
3   ❏ avoid use of contact lenses

A   ❏ 1, 2, 3
B   ❏ 1, 2 only
C   ❏ 2, 3 only
D   ❏ 1 only
E   ❏ 3 only

Q99   Eye drops:

1   ❏ are generally instilled into the pocket formed by gently pulling down the lower eyelid
2   ❏ the eye should be kept closed for as long as possible after application
3   ❏ the closure time is preferably 1–2 minutes

A   ❏ 1, 2, 3
B   ❏ 1, 2 only
C   ❏ 2, 3 only
D   ❏ 1 only
E   ❏ 3 only

Q100 Chloramphenicol eye drops:

1   ❏ are sterile before opening
2   ❏ contain a preservative
3   ❏ are available in 30 mL containers

A   ❏ 1, 2, 3
B   ❏ 1, 2 only
C   ❏ 2, 3 only
D   ❏ 1 only
E   ❏ 3 only

Test 5

Answers

A1   C

First-line treatment in upper respiratory tract infections includes the use of penicillins, cephalosporins and macrolides. Patients who are allergic to penicillins tend to be cross-sensitive to cephalosporins, so are given macrolides such as clarithromycin.

A2   E

The opioid analgesics, such as codeine, tramadol and fentanyl may cause drowsiness. Sumatriptan, which is a serotonin agonist, also tends to cause drowsiness. Modern non-steroidal anti-inflammatory drugs, such as diclofenac, do not cause drowsiness.

A3   C

Extemporaneous preparations, such as creams that are prepared in the pharmacy, have an expiry date of 4 weeks. The creams can be stored at room temperature.

A4   A

Statins, such as fluvastatin, may cause myalgia as a sign of myopathy. Patients are advised to report myalgia immediately.

A5   C

Diabetic patients are advised to carry sweets as a source of sugar in case of a hypoglycaemic reaction.

A6   B

A solution of 1 g of sodium chloride in 100 mL water makes up a 1% w/v solution.

A7 C

Thiazide diuretics act on the beginning of the distal convoluted tubule by inhibiting sodium re-absorption. Thiazide diuretics are indicated in hypertension, and at higher doses to relieve oedema caused by heart failure. Thiazide diuretics lead to hyponatraemia and hypokalaemia. They may cause hypercalcaemia and are therefore avoided in patients with this condition.

A8 B

Concomitant intake of alcohol and metronidazole is potentially dangerous, leading to a disulfiram-like type reaction characterised by intense vasodilatation, throbbing headache, tachycardia and sweating which can lead to death.

A9 D

High concentrations of vitamin A in pregnancy tend to be teratogenic leading to birth defects. Hence vitamin A is contraindicated in pregnancy.

A10 C

Itraconazole is a triazole antifungal, which increases the plasma concentration of digoxin, hence increasing the risk of digoxin toxicity.

A11 A

A patient needs to take five prednisolone 5 mg tablets in a day to make up a daily 25 mg dose. For a five-day supply the patient must be dispensed with 25 prednisolone 5 mg tablets.

A12 E

Metformin is an oral hypoglycaemic agent classified as a biguanide. Metformin decreases gluconeogenesis and increases peripheral utilisation of glucose. Metformin may be used in combination with sulphonylureas. Glibenclamide and chlorpropamide are long-acting sulphonylureas whereas gliclazide, glimepiride and tolbutamide are short-acting and are therefore less likely to be associated with hypoglycaemic attacks.

A13 C

The amount of intravenous fluid administered by noon (240 minutes) is 666 mL (1000 × 240/360). The amount of fluid administered between noon and midnight is 1000 mL. The total amount of intravenous fluid administered between 8.00 am and midnight is 1666 mL.

A14 B

Topical preparations for the treatment of acne include the use of azelaic acid, salicylic acid, benzoyl peroxide and triclosan. Clindamycin is an antibacterial preparation available for use in the treatment of acne both topically and systemically.

A15 D

Codeine, dextromethorphan and pholcodine are opioid cough suppressants indicated for dry cough. Sedating antihistamines, such as diphenhydramine, tend to have an antitussive action as well. Vitamin C is not used in the management of cough but may be used as a prophylaxis against colds.

A16 B

Amitriptyline is a tricyclic antidepressant.

A17 D

The dose 0.25 g is equivalent to 250 mg (half the 500 mg Naproxen tablet). The patient requires 14 doses of 250 mg Naproxen tablets and therefore seven 500 mg Naproxen tablets.

A18 B

The dose for this child is 6250 µg or 6.25 mg (250 µg × 25 kg).

A19   A

Tapeworm infections are caused by *Taenia solium*. Tinea pedis causes the fungal infection known as athlete's foot, *Yersinia pestis* is implicated in plague, *Candida albicans* is responsible for candidiasis while *Chlamydia trachomitis* causes eye infections.

A20   D

Body mass index is calculated by the formula weight in kg/(height in metres)^2. The body mass index for this patient is 28, i.e. $85/(1.74)^2$.

A21   B

Scabies is a skin infection caused by mites. Septicaemia occurs when bacterial microorganisms or their toxins enter the bloodstream. Endocarditis refers to bacterial infections of the endocardium. Peritonitis occurs when bacterial microorganisms infect the peritoneum. Shighellosis refers to infections caused by the *Shighella* bacteria.

A22   A

Salbutamol is a selective beta$_2$-receptor agonist indicated in the management of asthma as a bronchodilator relieving acute attacks. It may be used in combination with inhaled corticosteroids such as beclometasone. Salbutamol acts within a few minutes and tends to be short-acting, unlike salmeterol. Side-effects of salbutamol include tachycardia and palpitations. It does not cause drowsiness and does not precipitate oral candidiasis. Inhaled corticosteroids may precipitate oral candidiasis.

A23   E

Dysuria refers to difficult or painful urination. Dysuria generally indicates urinary tract infections. Symptoms of hyperglycaemia include polyuria (excretion of abnormally large quantity of urine), polydipsia (excessive thirst), visual disturbances, ketonuria and weakness.

A24   A

Ergotamine is an ergot alkaloid indicated for the treatment of migraine. It is contraindicated in hepatic impairment. Side-effects of ergotamine include tingling of extremities, caused by peripheral vasodilation and muscular cramps. Sumatriptan is a serotonin ($5HT_1$) agonist also indicated for the treatment of migraine. The value of ergotamine in the management of migraine is limited because of the occurrence of side-effects, including nausea and vomiting. It does not have any anti-emetic properties.

A25   E

Chlorpromazine is an aliphatic phenothiazine antipsychotic used in schizophrenia and which may exacerbate parkinsonism. Co-careldopa is a combination of levodopa and the peripheral dopa-decarboxylase inhibitor, carbidopa. Co-careldopa, amantadine, entacapone and bromocriptine are all indicated in the management of parkinsonism.

A26   A

Oxytocin is administered by slow intravenous infusion for labour induction.

A27   D

Sumatriptan is a serotonin ($5HT_1$) agonist, which does not cause dry mouth. Trihexyphenidyl, cinnarizine, imipramine and orphenadrine all tend to cause antimuscarinic side-effects, including dry mouth, constipation, blurred vision and urinary retention.

A28   E

The infusion is delivering 500 mL in 240 minutes (60 minutes $\times$ 4 hours) and 1 mL is delivered in 0.48 minute (240/500). Since the infusion set delivers 10 drops/mL, 10 drops are delivered in 0.48 minute and 21 drops are delivered per minute (10/0.48).

A29   B

Furuncles (boils) are caused by staphylococci. Fusidic acid is very effective against boils. Hydrocortisone is a low-potency corticosteroid. Aciclovir (antiviral) is indicated for the treatment and prophylaxis of herpes infections. Promethazine is an antihistamine cream and zinc oxide acts as a barrier when used in creams.

A30   E

Corticosteroids are unlikely to cause sensitisation. Both antihistamines (mepyramine) and local anaesthetics (prilocaine, benzocaine, lidocaine) may lead to sensitisation.

A31   D

Sodium chloride 0.9% is safe and effective in relieving rhinorrhoea. It is safer to use in children than topical nasal decongestants (xylometazoline), which are to be avoided in children under 6 years as the latter are more likely are cause side-effects (such as effects on sleep or hallucinations). Budesonide spray is used for allergic conditions and is not normally used in paediatric patients. Benzydamine spray is a throat spray intended to relieve pain in the throat. Mupirocin is indicated for staphylococcal infections.

A32   E

Magnesium hydroxide is a laxative and is not a constituent of oral rehydration salts, which tend to be recommended for use in diarrhoea, to avoid dehydration. Sodium chloride, glucose, potassium chloride and sodium citrate are required to maintain a proper electrolyte balance and are included in oral rehydration salts.

A33   D

Carbocisteine is classified as a mucolytic as it reduces sputum viscosity and aids its elimination. Carbocisteine is therefore indicated for use in chesty cough. Pholcodine, dextromethorphan and the sedating antihistamines, such as promethazine and chlorphenamine, are indicated in dry cough as cough suppressants.

A34 C

Diclofenac (a non-steroidal anti-inflammatory drug) is marketed as Voltarol oral slow-release formulations.

A35 C

Bumetanide is a loop diuretic indicated in oedema. Common side-effects of loop diuretics include hypokalaemia, hyponatraemia, hypotension and gout.

A36 C

Baclofen is a skeletal muscle relaxant.

A37 B

Aluminium chloride is a potent antiperspirant indicated for hyperhidrosis, particularly of the feet.

A38 B

Docusate sodium is a preparation used for softening ear wax before removal. Hydrocortisone is a corticosteroid, whereas gentamicin, neomycin and clioquinol are antibacterial agents. Otitis externa may be managed by the use of antibacterial preparations used alone or in combination with topical corticosteroids.

A39 B

Symptoms of hepatic failure include accumulation of fluid in the abdomen and lower body leading to ascites, weight loss, muscle wasting, jaundice and anaemia.

A40 C

Peripheral neuropathy is a complication of rheumatoid arthritis.

A41   E

Paget's disease may predispose to secondary osteoarthritis.

A42   C

PMH refers to past medical history.

A43   A

NIDDM refers to non-insulin dependent diabetes mellitus.

A44   E

CAPD refers to continuous ambulatory peritoneal dialysis.

A45   D

Choline salicylate provides analgesic action and is indicated in toothache.

A46   C

Nystatin is a polyene antifungal, which may be used orally for the treatment of intestinal candidiasis.

A47   E

Chlorhexidine is an antiseptic mouthwash that inhibits plaque formation on the teeth.

A48   E

Chlorhexidine may cause brown staining of the teeth and therefore patients are advised not to use chlorhexidine on a long-term basis.

A49   E

Fluticasone is a potent corticosteroid that is available as a nasal spray indicated in allergic rhinitis (hay fever) and as an inhaler used in asthma.

A50   A

Prednisolone is a corticosteroid that may be used orally for long-term disease suppression.

A51   D

Proprietary preparations of hydrocortisone for skin administration present a low-potency corticosteroid for topical skin administration.

A52   D

Prolonged febrile convulsions can be treated by administration of diazepam (benzodiazepine) as a slow intravenous infusion or rectally.

A53   B

Glaucoma is characterised by an increase in intraocular pressure. Clinical features of glaucoma include ocular pain, visual disturbances, headache and sometimes nausea and vomiting.

A54   B

Predisposing factors for low back pain include osteoporosis, trauma and pregnancy.

A55   C

Loperamide is an antimotility drug indicated for diarrhoea. Side-effects of loperamide include skin reactions and abdominal cramps.

A56   B

Sympathomimetics, such as dobutamine and isoprenaline, mimic the sympathetic system. Orphenadrine is an antimuscarinic drug acting as an antagonist to the parasympathetic system.

A57   B

Prophylaxis of angina may be managed by beta-adrenoceptor blockers, such as atenolol, and long-acting nitrates, such as isosorbide dinitrate. Digoxin is a cardiac glycoside that increases the force of myocardial contraction and reduces the conductivity of the heart. Digoxin is indicated as a positive inotrope in heart failure and as an anti-arrhythmic drug in atrial fibrillation.

A58   B

Angiotensin-converting enzyme inhibitors are indicated for use in hypertension and heart failure. Angiotensin-converting enzyme inhibitors have no use in the management of arrhythmias.

A59   E

Treatment of an acute attack of gout is managed by non-steroidal anti-inflammatory drugs, such as naproxen. Drugs such as allopurinol and other uricosurics are not indicated for the treatment of an acute attack of gout as they may prolong the attack. Allopurinol is indicated for prophylaxis of gout and is used on a long-term basis. Indapamide is a thiazide diuretic, which may precipitate an acute attack of gout.

A60   D

Gentamicin is an aminoglycoside active against some Gram-positive bacteria and many Gram-negative bacteria. Gentamicin is inactive against anaerobes. Monitoring of the renal function is important when administering gentamicin.

A61   E

Patient information leaflets are intended to provide information about the medicine to the patient. The leaflets are produced for many medicines whether presented as original packs or patient packs. For medicines presented in bulk dispensing packs, the manufacturer may supply additional copies of the leaflet. Within the European Union, Directive 92/27/EEC outlines the contents of patient information leaflets and the use of the rINN is required.

A62   B

Tinnitus is the perception of sound, such as buzzing, hissing or pulsating noises, in the ears. Tinnitus may be caused by aspirin overdosage, furosemide or gentamicin toxicity. Tinnitus may also be an accompanying symptom of senile deafness, otosclerosis and Meniere's disease.

A63   A

Adverse drug reactions may be characterised by urticaria, fever or maculopapular rashes.

A64   B

Selective serotonin re-uptake inhibitors (SSRIs) and tricyclic antidepressants are equally effective. However, SSRIs tend to have fewer antimuscarinic side-effects and are less cardiotoxic in case of overdosage. SSRIs tend to cause gastrointestinal side-effects. Both SSRIs and tricylic antidepressants exhibit a time lag before the action of the antidepressants becomes effective.

A65   B

Decreased mobility or immobility and incontinence are risk factors for the development of pressure ulcers. The use of appropriate barrier skin creams may protect against the development of pressure sores, especially in bed-ridden patients.

A66   A

Clinical trials involve different phases of studies of the drug. The aim of clinical trials is to assess safety and efficacy of a drug in humans. Clinical trials must follow good clinical practice guidelines.

A67   D

Iron salts should always be administered by mouth unless there are good reasons for using another route. Ferrous salts are better absorbed than ferric salts. Iron salts may cause gastrointestinal disturbances and are therefore administered after food.

A68   D

Amenorrhoea, which refers to the absence of menstruation, is managed by the administration of progestogen components such as dydrogesterone. Non-steroidal anti-inflammatory drugs are indicated in premenstrual tension. Iron supplements are indicated in menorrhagia (abnormal heavy menstruation).

A69   E

One of the main disadvantages of depot parenteral preparations is that administration of these preparations may not be acceptable to the patient. The depot preparation requires a lower dosing frequency when compared with other dosage forms.

A70   B

Cetirizine is a non-sedating antihistamine drug that may be used for symptomatic relief in allergic rhinitis (hay fever) as it reduces rhinorrhoea and sneezing. Fexofenadine is an active metabolite of terfenadine (another antihistamine).

A71   B

Rubefacients act by counter-irritation produced as a result of local vasodilation, resulting in a warm sensation that masks the pain. Counter-irritants should not be applied on broken skin or before or after taking a hot shower. Examples of counter-irritants include salicylates, nicotinates, capsicum, menthol and camphor. Ketoprofen is an example of a non-steroidal anti-inflammatory drug that is available as a topical preparation indicated in painful musculoskeletal conditions.

A72 E

Thyroxine (levothyroxine) is indicated in hypothyroidism as a maintenance therapy on a long-term basis. The initial dose must not exceed 100 µg. The usual maintenance dose is 100–200 µg. The dose is decreased in elderly patients. Thyroxine must be taken in the morning.

A73 E

Emollients are useful in eczema as they soothe, smooth and hydrate the skin. The action of emollients tends to be short-lived and therefore they need to be applied frequently.

A74 B

Ketoconazole and coal tar are available as preparations intended for scalp application and are indicated against dandruff and psoriasis or chronic atopic eczema respectively.

A75 B

Babies under 3 months with diarrhoea and infants under 1 year presenting with diarrhoea that persists for more than 24 hours require referral. Diarrhoea accompanied by vomiting does not usually warrant referral unless the vomiting or diarrhoea are severe.

A76 C

Athlete's foot, tinea pedis, is a condition caused by a fungus. Management of athlete's foot lies with the use of antifungal preparations such as clotrimazole (an imidazole antifungal) and tolnaftate. Salicylic acid is a keratolytic agent indicated for use in treatment of corns, calluses and warts.

A77 C

Viral meningitis refers to inflammation of the meninges. It is characterised by headache, neck stiffness and may be accompanied by fever. Lumbar puncture is required to differentiate between bacterial meningitis and viral meningitis.

Viral meningitis, unlike bacterial meningitis, resolves spontaneously and is not life threatening.

A78   D

Magnesium salts are powerful osmotic laxatives, which are useful when rapid evacuation is required and are therefore indicated for bowel cleansing prior to examination of the gastrointestinal tract or before surgery. Glycerin is a stimulant laxative that acts through an irritant action. Ispaghula husk is a bulk-forming laxative, which may be used on a long-term basis but does not bring about a rapid bowel cleansing.

A79   A

Cough may be an accompanying symptom of respiratory tract infections. It is associated with smoking and may be an indication of lung cancer.

A80   B

During pregnancy, a well-balanced diet consisting of starch, fibre, vitamins and minerals is essential. Foods rich in sugar, fats and refined carbohydrates must be limited.

A81   D

Medium-textured brushes are best in removing plaque without causing gingival trauma, as may occur with the hard-texture brushes.

A82   E

Exercise in not contraindicated in controlled angina. However, patients are advised to carry with them glyceryl trinitrate. Swimming is not associated with triggering of exercise-induced asthma.

A83   C

Support bandages help brace an injured area during movement but do not reduce risk of infections.

A84 B

Calamine lotion provides a cooling effect that soothes the skin and may be applied after a jellyfish sting. Jellyfish release histamine, which results in erythema and itchiness.

A85 A

Co-amoxiclav is a combination of amoxicillin (the beta-lactam penicillin) and clavulanic acid, a beta-lactamase inhibitor.

A86 A

Co-amoxiclav suspension should be reconstituted with mineral water before dispensing. The parent must be advised to shake the bottle well before use and to administer to the child 5 mL twice daily.

A87 A

The dose of paracetamol suppositories for a 5-year-old child is 125–250 mg four times daily.

A88 B

The parent may be advised to check body temperature, thereby monitoring fever and to keep the child well hydrated. Co-amoxiclav suspension has to be continued for 7 days.

A89 B

Paracetamol suppositories may have been preferred to the oral dosage form, either because the patient is reluctant to take the medication or because the patient is vomiting.

A90–92

Cystitis is a condition where urinary tract bacterial infection is presented. Products recommended as first-line of treatment include amoxicillin, oral cephalosporin, trimethoprim or nitrofurantoin. Doxycycline is a tetracycline antibacterial agent whereas itraconazole is an antifungal agent.

A90   1

A91   2

A92   3

A93   B

Paracetamol is indicated as an anti-pyretic and may be safely administered in a patient on warfarin. A topical nasal decongestant is effective for rhinorrhoea (runny nose) and would not interfere with warfarin. Altering the dose of warfarin is only recommended on the basis of results of international normalised ratio (INR) levels.

A94   E

The patient would be advised to seek medical advice if the condition gets worse, as antibacterial agents may be required.

A95   B

Conjunctivitis is inflammation of the conjunctiva. Conjunctivitis may be bacterial, in which case it is accompanied by a purulent discharge, viral or allergic in origin. Generally symptoms include erythema and itchiness.

A96   D

Chloramphenicol is a broad-spectrum antibiotic indicated for superficial eye infections. Products containing corticosteroids should not be used in undiagnosed 'red eye' since the administration of the corticosteroid may remove the symptoms although the condition may not be addressed.

A97   D

Chloramphenicol eye preparations may cause transient stinging as with any other eye preparation. Agranulocytosis refers to deficiency in neutrophils. Photophobia refers to abnormal intolerance to light.

A98   A

All patients with eye infections are advised to avoid wearing contact lenses. In this case the patient must also be advised to apply the drops in the morning and at midday and to apply the ointment at night.

A99   A

Patients using eye drops are advised to pull down the lower eye lid gently and instil the drops in the pocket formed without touching the dropper with the eyelid. The patient must be advised to keep the eyes closed for as long as possible, closure time being at least 1–2 minutes.

A100   B

All eye drops, including chloramphenicol, are sterile before opening and must be discarded within 4 weeks of opening. Eye drops contain a preservative and are available in small-volume containers (10 mL).

Test 6

Questions

Questions 1–38

Directions: Each of the questions or incomplete statements is followed by five suggested answers. Select the best answer in each case.

Q1 Which one of the following is suitable for the management of lower urinary tract infection in a pregnant woman?

A ❑ co-trimoxazole
B ❑ ciprofloxacin
C ❑ aztreonam
D ❑ co-amoxiclav
E ❑ doxycycline

Q2 For which of the following drugs should the label p.c. be used:

A ❑ salbutamol
B ❑ tetracycline
C ❑ prednisolone
D ❑ codeine
E ❑ glyceryl trinitrate

Q3 The maximum volume that should be given as a single intramuscular injection at one site is:

A ❑ 20 mL
B ❑ 0.1 mL
C ❑ 1.0 mL
D ❑ 5 mL
E ❑ 2 mL

Q4   A 53-year-old administrative person being treated for hypertension
with atenolol 100 mg once daily may report:

    A   ❑ dry mouth
    B   ❑ palpitations
    C   ❑ difficulty with micturition
    D   ❑ urticaria
    E   ❑ fatigue

Q5   Non-pharmacological methods that lower blood pressure include all
EXCEPT:

    A   ❑ decreasing alcohol consumption
    B   ❑ relaxation techniques
    C   ❑ regular exercise
    D   ❑ stopping smoking
    E   ❑ taking small, frequent meals

Q6   A 1% w/v solution of a local anaesthetic contains:

    A   ❑ 1 mg in 100 mL
    B   ❑ 1 g in 100 mL
    C   ❑ 10 mg in 1 mL
    D   ❑ 1 g in 1 mL
    E   ❑ 100 mg in 100 mL

Q7   Phenothiazines should usually be avoided in patients with:

    A   ❑ hypertension
    B   ❑ anxiety
    C   ❑ depression
    D   ❑ closed-angle glaucoma
    E   ❑ insomnia

Q8   Which of the following does not alter a patient's insulin requirements?

A   ❑   pregnancy
B   ❑   major surgery
C   ❑   proton pump inhibitors
D   ❑   severe infection
E   ❑   food intake patterns

Q9   Which of these drugs cannot be used to induce labour or to cause the uterus to contract after delivery?

A   ❑   ritodrine
B   ❑   dinoprostone
C   ❑   ergometrine
D   ❑   oxytocin
E   ❑   carboprost

Q10   A patient is being started on amiloride/hydrochlorthiazide tablets. Which drug may interact with the diuretic?

A   ❑   salbutamol
B   ❑   enalapril
C   ❑   diazepam
D   ❑   senna
E   ❑   atenolol

Q11   Which normal tissue is especially liable to be damaged by cytotoxic drugs?

A   ❑   brain
B   ❑   cartilage
C   ❑   muscle
D   ❑   intestinal mucosa
E   ❑   bone

Q12   All of the following are antibacterial agents classified as amino-glycosides EXCEPT:

A   ❏ gentamicin
B   ❏ tobramycin
C   ❏ azithromycin
D   ❏ amikacin
E   ❏ kanamycin

Q13   Quoting 50 378.9576 to three significant figures reads:

A   ❏ 503
B   ❏ 50 300
C   ❏ 50 400
D   ❏ 50 378.957
E   ❏ 50 378.958

Q14   Which anti-infective preparation is available only as a topical dosage form?

A   ❏ ketoconazole
B   ❏ terbinafine
C   ❏ mupirocin
D   ❏ fusidic acid
E   ❏ griseofulvin

Q15   Which of the following is not a nasal decongestant?

A   ❏ phenylpropanolamine
B   ❏ triprolidine
C   ❏ pseudoephedrine
D   ❏ phenylephrine
E   ❏ oxymetazoline

Q16 Calculate the weight in grams of 1 mole sulphate in calcium sulphate (relative atomic mass of calcium = 40.08; sulphur = 32.07; oxygen = 16.00):

A ❏ 48
B ❏ 64
C ❏ 96
D ❏ 136
E ❏ 144

Q17 Calculate the dose of domperidone suspension to be administered to a patient if the paediatric dosing regimen is listed as 2.5 mg/ 10 kg three times daily. The patient weighs 30 kg. Domperidone suspension contains 1 mg of domperidone per mL.

A ❏ 2.5 mL t.d.s.
B ❏ 5 mL t.d.s.
C ❏ 1 mL t.d.s.
D ❏ 75 mL t.d.s.
E ❏ 7.5 mL t.d.s.

Q18 The adult intravenous dose of gentamicin is 2 mg/kg every 8 hours. How many milligrams will a 65 kg patient receive daily?

A ❏ 130 mg
B ❏ 1040 mg
C ❏ 390 mg
D ❏ 16 mg
E ❏ 520 mg

Q19 Clotrimazole is indicated to treat infections caused by:

A ❏ *Candida albicans*
B ❏ *Chlamydia trachomatis*
C ❏ *Neisseria gonorrhoea*
D ❏ *Staphylcoccus aureus*
E ❏ *Streptococcus pneumoniae*

Q20   Which over-the-counter product is indicated for acute constipation?

A   ❏   loperamide
B   ❏   ispaghula husk
C   ❏   kaolin and morphine
D   ❏   lactulose
E   ❏   bisacodyl

Q21   The rubella virus has the most serious effect on:

A   ❏   an elderly patient
B   ❏   a pregnant woman
C   ❏   a newborn infant
D   ❏   a first-trimester fetus
E   ❏   an adolescent girl

Q22   Pharmacological effects of calcium-channel blocking agents may include:

A   ❏   venoconstriction
B   ❏   arteriodilatation
C   ❏   hypertension
D   ❏   positive inotropic effect
E   ❏   increased conduction at the sinoatrial and atrioventricular nodes

Q23   Characteristic symptoms of peptic ulcer disease include all EXCEPT:

A   ❏   diffuse abdominal pain
B   ❏   pain relief by food
C   ❏   pain during the night
D   ❏   pain relieved by antacids
E   ❏   occasional vomiting

Q24   Metoclopramide:

   A   ❑ is a dopamine agonist
   B   ❑ is not associated with extrapyramidal symptoms
   C   ❑ may be used for prophylaxis of travel sickness
   D   ❑ adult daily dose is 30 mg
   E   ❑ increases oesophageal sphincter contraction

Q25   Drugs used in the treatment of prophylaxis of angina include all EXCEPT:

   A   ❑ glyceryl trinitrate
   B   ❑ isosorbide dinitrate
   C   ❑ nifedipine
   D   ❑ atenolol
   E   ❑ losartan

Q26   Carbamazepine is used in the treatment of:

   A   ❑ trigeminal neuralgia
   B   ❑ parkinsonism
   C   ❑ hyperthyroidism
   D   ❑ hypothyroidism
   E   ❑ dementia

Q27   Which of the following drugs is not liable to cause constipation?

   A   ❑ codeine
   B   ❑ amitriptyline
   C   ❑ orphenadrine
   D   ❑ senna
   E   ❑ tramadol

Q28 The amount in grams of potassium permanganate required to prepare 25 mL of a 1 in 55 solution is:

A ☐ 0.04
B ☐ 0.45
C ☐ 1
D ☐ 2.2
E ☐ 4.5

Q29 Which of the following is of value in the management of eczema?

A ☐ fatty cream base
B ☐ podophyllum
C ☐ lidocaine
D ☐ calcipotriol
E ☐ clindamycin

Q30 Which one of the following drugs is likely to cause photosensitivity?

A ☐ amiodarone
B ☐ ferrous sulphate
C ☐ digoxin
D ☐ isosorbide dinitrate
E ☐ propranolol

Q31 A mother comes to the pharmacy with her 3-year-old son who has a cough. Which of the following list of symptoms is most likely to indicate an allergy?

A ☐ fever
B ☐ chesty cough
C ☐ rhinorrhoea
D ☐ headache
E ☐ malaise

Q32   Constituents of calamine lotion BP include calamine and:

A   ❑ aluminium oxide
B   ❑ sodium chloride
C   ❑ zinc oxide
D   ❑ magnesium hydroxide
E   ❑ calcium carbonate

Q33   In gastro-oesophageal reflux disease, which of the following constituents of antacids may be particularly useful:

A   ❑ aluminium hydroxide
B   ❑ sodium alginate
C   ❑ chloroform water
D   ❑ sucrose
E   ❑ lactose

Q34   For which of the following drugs are there significant differences in bioavailability after oral administration:

A   ❑ propranolol
B   ❑ ampicillin
C   ❑ theophylline
D   ❑ erythromycin
E   ❑ paroxetine

Q35   Common side-effects of itraconazole include all EXCEPT:

A   ❑ nausea
B   ❑ palpitations
C   ❑ dizziness
D   ❑ headache
E   ❑ abdominal pain

Q36   Dextromethorphan:

A   ❏ is an opioid antitussive
B   ❏ is an analgesic
C   ❏ has antipyretic effects
D   ❏ is recommended for use in children under 2 years of age
E   ❏ causes diarrhoea as a side-effect

Q37   Topical products for removal of corns and calluses may contain salicylic acid as a (an):

A   ❏ keratolytic agent
B   ❏ bactericidal agent
C   ❏ emollient
D   ❏ local anaesthetic
E   ❏ anhidrotic agent

Q38   Agents that could be recommended for dandruff include all EXCEPT:

A   ❏ selenium sulphide
B   ❏ coal tar
C   ❏ ketoconazole
D   ❏ permethrin
E   ❏ salicylic acid

Questions 39–51

Directions: Each group of questions below consists of five lettered
headings followed by a list of numbered questions. For
each numbered question select the one heading that is
most closely related to it. Each heading may be used once,
more than once, or not at all.

Questions 39–41 concern the following conditions:

A ❑ Diabetes
B ❑ Raised intracranial pressure
C ❑ Pregnancy
D ❑ Diverticulitis
E ❑ Oral thrush

Select, from A to E, which one of the above:

Q39 could be a cause of lower gastrointestinal bleeding

Q40 could be a cause of early morning headache

Q41 could be a cause of early morning vomiting

Questions 42–44 concern the following amino acids:

A ❑ tyrosine
B ❑ serine
C ❑ histidine
D ❑ tryptophan
E ❑ hydroxyproline

Select, from A to E, the amino acid from which each of the following neurotransmitters is synthesised:

Q42 noradrenaline

Q43 serotonin

Q44 histamine

Questions 45–48 concern the following drugs:

A ❑ folic acid
B ❑ calcium
C ❑ riboflavin
D ❑ magnesium
E ❑ retinol

Select, from A to E, which one of the above:

Q45   is vitamin B_2

Q46   may be found in combination with bisphosphonates

Q47   is used in combination therapy with methotrexate

Q48   is contraindicated during pregnancy

Questions 49–51 concern the following drugs:

A ❑ piperacillin
B ❑ penicillin V
C ❑ penicillin G
D ❑ ampicillin
E ❑ flucloxacillin

Select, from A to E, which one of the above:

Q49   is particularly active against *Pseudomonas aeruginosa*

Q50   is inactivated by gastric acid

Q51   is an oral penicillin that is resistant to beta-lactamase

Questions 52–79

Directions: For each of the questions below, ONE or MORE of the responses is (are) correct. Decide which of the responses is (are) correct. Then choose:

A   ❑ if 1, 2 and 3 are correct
B   ❑ if 1 and 2 only are correct
C   ❑ if 2 and 3 only are correct
D   ❑ if 1 only is correct
E   ❑ if 3 only is correct

Directions summarised				
A	B	C	D	E
1, 2, 3	1, 2 only	2, 3 only	1 only	3 only

Q52   Which of the following is (are) recognised treatments for Crohn's disease?

1   ❑ oral lactulose
2   ❑ oral corticosteroids
3   ❑ oral sulfasalazine

Q53   Clinical features of hyperthyroidism include:

1   ❑ palpitations
2   ❑ tremor
3   ❑ weight gain

Q54   Predisposing factors for osteoporosis include:

1   ❑ excessive exercise
2   ❑ obesity
3   ❑ advanced age

Q55   Side-effects of application of topical steroids to the skin include:

1   ❏   thickening of the skin
2   ❏   spread of local skin infection
3   ❏   striae

Q56   Fibrinolytic agents include:

1   ❏   tranexamic acid
2   ❏   urokinase
3   ❏   alteplase

Q57   Drugs useful in the prophylaxis of migraine include:

1   ❏   ergotamine
2   ❏   amitriptyline
3   ❏   propranolol

Q58   Therapeutic uses of benzodiazepines include:

1   ❏   alcohol withdrawal
2   ❏   status epilepticus
3   ❏   obsessive compulsive disorder

Q59   Treatment of Parkinson's disease includes:

1   ❏   bromocriptine
2   ❏   orphenadrine
3   ❏   moclobemide

Q60   Doxycycline:

1   ❏   is a bacteriostatic
2   ❏   is a broad-spectrum antibacterial drug
3   ❏   is effective against chlamydiae

Q61   Which of the following are legal requirements in a prescription?

1   ❑ prescription must be dated
2   ❑ prescriber's signature
3   ❑ price of medication

Q62   Tardive dyskinesia:

1   ❑ is particularly prone to occur in the older patient
2   ❑ occurs at a higher frequency with clozapine compared with haloperidol
3   ❑ is due to reduced dopamine activity

Q63   Causes of acute inflammation include:

1   ❑ bacterial infection
2   ❑ trauma
3   ❑ cardiac arrhythmias

Q64   Advantages of the combined oral contraceptives over the progestogen-only contraceptives are that they are:

1   ❑ suitable for breast-feeding women
2   ❑ less likely to cause deep vein thrombosis
3   ❑ less likely to be associated with irregular vaginal bleeding

Q65   Causes of conjunctivitis include:

1   ❑ viral infection
2   ❑ bacterial infection
3   ❑ chlamydiae infection

Q66   Containers used for dispensing medicines should:

1   ❑ always be glass containers
2   ❑ be cleaned with alcohol before use
3   ❑ be labelled accordingly

Q67 Clarithromycin:

1 ❏ cannot be prescribed in conjunction with amoxicillin
2 ❏ has a shorter half-life than erythromycin
3 ❏ is used in *Helicobacter pylori* eradication regimens

Q68 Which of the following drugs is likely to be prescribed routinely in the treatment of asthma?

1 ❏ amoxicillin
2 ❏ codeine
3 ❏ budesonide

Q69 Disadvantages of inhaled steroids in asthma therapy include:

1 ❏ hoarseness
2 ❏ oral candidiasis
3 ❏ adrenal suppression

Q70 Lactulose:

1 ❏ acts within 8 hours
2 ❏ acts as an osmotic laxative
3 ❏ may cause abdominal discomfort

Q71 Hormone replacement therapy:

1 ❏ provides relief from vasomotor symptoms
2 ❏ decreases risk of osteoporosis
3 ❏ increases risk of cardiovascular disease

Q72 Indometacin:

1 ❏ has a superior anti-inflammatory action compared with ibuprofen
2 ❏ rectal administration prevents gastrointestinal tract adverse effects
3 ❏ stimulates cyclo-oxygenase

Q73   Magnesium-containing antacids:

1   ❏ should be used with caution in renal impairment
2   ❏ may cause constipation
3   ❏ should not be administered at the same time as aluminium salts

Q74   Which preparations are available for administration to the eye?

1   ❏ dexamethasone
2   ❏ betamethasone
3   ❏ docusate sodium

Q75   Accompanying conditions to foot disorders that indicate referral include:

1   ❏ fungal infections
2   ❏ rashes
3   ❏ toenail involvement

Q76 The serum drug concentration:

1   ❏ is always equal to the effect
2   ❏ is always equivalent to in-vitro tests
3   ❏ following oral dosing may be affected by the drug's distribution pathways

Q77   Amenorrhoea is associated with:

1   ❏ anorexia nervosa
2   ❏ polycystic ovary syndrome
3   ❏ congenital adrenal hyperplasia

Q78   Which of the following drugs would be effective in the treatment of an acute attack of mania?

1   ❏ lithium
2   ❏ haloperidol
3   ❏ flupentixol

Q79 Back pain may be associated with:

1 ❑ osteomalacia
2 ❑ osteoporosis
3 ❑ pregnancy

Questions 80–90

Directions: The following questions consist of a first statement followed by a second statement. Decide whether the first statement is true or false. Decide whether the second statement is true or false. Then choose:

A ❑ if both statements are true and the second statement is a *correct explanation* of the first statement

B ❑ if both statements are true but the second statement *is NOT a correct explanation* of the first statement

C ❑ if the first statement is true but the second statement is false

D ❑ if the first statement is false but the second statement is true

E ❑ if both statements are false

Directions summarised			
	First statement	**Second statement**	
A	True	True	Second statement is a *correct explanation* of the first
B	True	True	Second statement is *NOT a correct explanation* of the first
C	True	False	
D	False	True	
E	False	False	

Q80 Lorazepam may be used for short-term relief of severe anxiety. Lorazepam is a short-acting benzodiazepine.

Q81 An ultrablock sunscreen preparation always has a sun protection factor of 30. Sunscreen preparations protect the skin from the damage associated with ultraviolet A (UVA).

Q82 A patient with prostatic hypertrophy who has a chesty cough could be advised to use carbocisteine syrup. Carbocisteine syrup does not contain antihistamine drugs.

Q83 Eye drops should be discarded after 4 weeks from opening. Eye drops do not contain a preservative.

Q84 When providing information to the patient, the pharmacist has to convey the information directed to the individual patient's needs. The pharmacist should adjust to the patient's age, personality, and educational background.

Q85 Methotrexate is an antimetabolite of folic acid and has immunosuppressant properties. Methotrexate may be used in Crohn's disease.

Q86 Patients with a suspected infarction should receive analgesics intravenously as soon as possible. Pain in myocardial infarction may cause adverse haemodynamic effects such as increases in blood pressure and heart rate.

Q87 Morphine should not be used for pain relief in myocardial infarction. Morphine may induce hypotension as a side-effect.

Q88 Anti-inflammatory doses of aspirin may cause tinnitus and deafness. These side-effects are symptoms of salicylate intoxication.

Q89   Indometacin is an indole acetic acid derivative that has a lower frequency of gastrointestinal side-effects compared with naproxen. Indometacin may cause headache and dizziness as side-effects.

Q90   Mebendazole is not suitable for women known to be pregnant. Mebendazole, which is a benzimidazole carbamate derivative, has shown toxicity in rats.

Questions 91–100

Directions: These questions involve cases. Read the prescription or case and answer the questions.

Questions 91–92: Use the prescription below

```
Patient's name:          . . . . . . . . . . . . . . . . . . . . . . .

Age: 29 years
Fluocinolone acetonide cream
Apply twice daily    m. 1 tube



Doctor's signature:    . . . . . . . . . . . . . . . . . . . . . . .
```

Q91   Fluocinolone could be described as:

A   ❏ a mild anti-inflammatory agent
B   ❏ a potent anti-inflammatory agent with anti-infective properties
C   ❏ a potent anti-inflammatory agent
D   ❏ an anti-infective agent
E   ❏ an analgesic agent

Q92   The patient could have:

1   ❏ urticaria
2   ❏ rosacea
3   ❏ dermatitis

A   ❏ 1, 2, 3
B   ❏ 1, 2 only
C   ❏ 2, 3 only
D   ❏ 1 only
E   ❏ 3 only

Questions 93–95: Use the patient profile below

Patient medication profile

Patient's name: . . . .

Age: 42 years
Allergies: none
Diagnosis: hyperthyroidism
Medication record: carbimazole 10 mg daily

The patient comes to the pharmacy complaining of sore throat, fever, malaise and dry eyes for the past 2 weeks.

Q93   What line of action would you follow?

1   ❏ dispense Uniflu preparation
2   ❏ dispense hypromellose eye drops
3   ❏ refer patient

A   ❏ 1, 2, 3
B   ❏ 1, 2 only
C   ❏ 2, 3 only
D   ❏ 1 only
E   ❏ 3 only

After a few days the patient returns with the following prescription:

Patient's name: . . . .

Cefuroxime tablets 250 mg
b.d.   m. 10

Doctor's signature: . . . .

Q94   Cefuroxime:

   1   ❑ is active against *Haemophilus influenzae*
   2   ❑ is a second-generation cephalosporin
   3   ❑ may cause nausea, vomiting and headache as side-effects

   A   ❑ 1, 2, 3
   B   ❑ 1, 2 only
   C   ❑ 2, 3 only
   D   ❑ 1 only
   E   ❑ 3 only

Q95   The patient is advised to:

   1   ❑ take cefuroxime tablets for 5 days
   2   ❑ stop carbimazole tablets when taking the antibacterial agent
   3   ❑ return to the pharmacy within 2 days of starting treatment

   A   ❑ 1, 2, 3
   B   ❑ 1, 2 only
   C   ❑ 2, 3 only
   D   ❑ 1 only
   E   ❑ 3 only

Questions 96–100:

Cilest is a combined hormonal contraceptive.

Put the following adverse effects in order of occurrence assigning 1 to the side-effect that occurs most commonly and 5 to the side-effect that occurs least commonly.

Q96   acne

Q97   fluid retention

Q98   nausea

Q99   reduced menstrual loss

Q100 photosensitivity

Test 6

Answers

A1 D

Co-amoxiclav containing the beta-lactam amoxicillin (penicillin) and the beta-lactamase inhibitor clavulanic acid can be safely administered during pregnancy. Co-trimoxazole is contraindicated in pregnancy because of a teratogenic effect. The use of ciprofloxacin (quinolone) in pregnancy is contraindicated because of possible arthropathy in weight-bearing joints of the fetus. Aztreonam (monocyclic beta-lactam antibiotic) is avoided in pregnancy. Doxycyline (tetracycline) is contraindicated because of deposition in the bones and teeth of the fetus.

A2 C

Prednisolone tablets must be taken after food to prevent any gastrointestinal irritation and bleeding associated with the systemic administration of steroids.

A3 D

The maximum volume of any substance that can be given as a single intra-muscular injection at one site is 5 mL.

A4 E

Common side-effects associated with beta-adrenoceptor blockers, such as atenolol, include fatigue, bradycardia, sleep disturbances, and peripheral vasoconstriction leading to coldness of extremities. Water-soluble beta-blockers, such as atenolol, are less likely to cause sleep disturbances and nightmares than lipid-soluble beta-blockers, such as propranolol.

A5 E

Regular exercise helps in lowering blood pressure especially in obese patients. A sedentary lifestyle is often implicated in cardiovascular disease, such as hypertension. Other non-pharmacological methods that help reduce blood pressure include decrease in sodium intake, moderation of alcohol consumption, avoiding stress and stopping smoking for smokers. Healthy food patterns should be followed but it is not necessary to advise patients to take small, frequent meals.

A6   B

A 1% w/v solution contains 1 g of the active ingredient in 100 mL of the solution.

A7   D

Phenothiazines tend to have antimuscarinic properties and are therefore contraindicated for use in patients with closed-angle glaucoma. Antimuscarinics are contraindicated in closed-angle glaucoma as they may worsen the condition.

A8   C

A patient's insulin requirements are altered during pregnancy, major surgery, severe infections and as a result of changes in food intake patterns. Proton pump inhibitors do not affect insulin requirements.

A9   A

Ritodrine relaxes the uterine muscle and is therefore indicated to prevent premature labour. Ergometrine, oxytocin and carboprost are all indicated to induce or augment labour by inducing uterine contractions and hence can be used to cause the uterus to contract after delivery. Dinoprostone is mostly used for the induction of labour.

A10   B

Amiloride is a potassium-sparing diuretic, whereas hydrochlorthiazide is a thiazide diuretic that causes loss of potassium. Enalapril is an angiotensin-converting enzyme inhibitor that retains potassium, thereby counteracting the loss of potassium caused by the thiazide diuretic.

A11   D

Cytotoxic drugs are most toxic to rapidly proliferating cells, such as the intestinal mucosa, mucous membranes, skin, hair and bone marrow, leading to nausea and vomiting, stomatitis, alopecia and bone marrow toxicity.

A12   C

Azithromycin is a macrolide having greater activity against Gram-negative organisms than erythromycin but lower activity against Gram-positive organisms. Gentamicin, tobramycin, amikacin and neomycin are aminoglycosides.

A13   C

Quoting 50 378.9576 to three significant figures reads 50 400.

A14   C

Mupirocin is an antibiotic agent available only for topical use. It is indicated for use in Gram-positive skin infections. Mupirocin should not be used for more than 10 days, to prevent the emergence of resistance.

A15   B

Triprolidine is an antihistamine. Phenylpropranolamine, pseudoephedrine, phenylephrine and oxymetazoline are nasal decongestants. Nasal decongestants administered systemically are often available in combination with an antihistamine.

A16   C

1 mole sulphate is equivalent to 96 g (32.07 + 16 × 4).

A17   E

The dose for a patient weighing 30 kg would be (2.5 mg × 3) 7.5 mg three times daily. Considering that domperidone suspension contains 1 mg of domperidone per 1 mL, the dose that must be administered is 7.5 mL three times daily.

A18   C

The dose for a patient weighing 65 kg would be (65 kg × 2 mg) 130 mg every 8 hours; hence the total daily dose would be 390 mg.

A19   A

Clotrimazole is an imidazole antifungal agent indicated for the treatment of fungal infections caused by *Candida albicans*. The administration of clotrimazole would be of no use in the treatment of infections caused by *Chlamydia trachomatis, Neisseria gonorrhoea, Staphylcoccus aureus* and *Streptococcus pneumoniae*.

A20   E

Bisacodyl is a stimulant laxative that does not take long to act and is therefore useful in acute constipation. The bulk-forming laxative ispaghula husk takes longer to act when compared with bisacodyl but is useful for long-term administration. Lactulose, which is an osmotic laxative, has a lag time of about 48 hours before onset of action. Loperamide and kaolin and morphine mixture are antidiarrhoeals used in acute diarrhoea.

A21   D

Rubella, also known as German measles, is caused by the rubella virus. Rubella contracted during pregnancy is dangerous to the fetus, especially in the first trimester and may lead to stillbirths, congenital malformations or abortion.

A22   B

Calcium-channel blockers interfere with the inward movement of calcium ions through the cell membrane channels. This results in reduction of myocardial contractility (hence negative inotropes), reduction of cardiac output and arteriolar vasodilatation. The dihydropyridine group, such as nifedipine and amlodipine, which may be used in the management of hypertension, are very effective as arterial vasodilators, whereas diltiazem and verapamil are very effective in reducing atrioventricular conduction.

A23   A

Localised upper abdominal pain is the most common symptom of peptic ulcer disease. The pain is relieved by antacids, proton pump inhibitors and H_2 antagonists. The pain may or may not be relieved by food and is often worse during the night. Peptic ulceration may be accompanied by occasional vomiting, anorexia and weight loss. Diffuse abdominal pain is not a characteristic symptom of peptic ulcer disease.

A24   D

Metoclopramide is a dopamine antagonist indicated as an anti-emetic in vomiting associated with gastrointestinal, hepatic and biliary disorders and in vomiting associated with cytotoxics and radiotherapy. Metoclopramide, which enhances gastric emptying, is not effective in motion sickness. The adult dose of metoclopramide is 10 mg three times daily. Metoclopramide, being a dopamine antagonist, may result in extrapyramidal symptoms, particularly in young adults.

A25   E

Losartan is an angiotensin II receptor antagonist indicated as an alternative to angiotensin-converting enzyme inhibitor drugs in the management of hypertension and heart failure. Treatment and prophylaxis of angina is managed by nitrates, such as glyceryl trinitrate and isosorbide dinitrate; and by beta-adrenoceptor blockers, such as atenolol and by calcium-channel blockers, such as long-acting nifedipine.

A26   A

Carbamazepine is an anti-epileptic, which may also be used in the treatment of trigeminal neuralgia. Monitoring of carbamazepine plasma concentrations is required if high doses are administered as carbamazepine tends to be an autoinducer, meaning that the half-life is shortened following repeated administration of the drug.

A27   D

One of the main side-effects of opioid analgesics, such as codeine and tramadol, is constipation. Amitriptyline (tricyclic antidepressant) and orphenadrine tend to have antimuscarinic properties, resulting in side-effects such as constipation. Senna is a stimulant laxative indicated in constipation.

A28   B

For a 1 in 55 solution, 1 g is dissolved in 55 mL. Therefore for 25 mL, 0.45 g is required (25/55).

A29   A

Eczema is managed by emollients and topical corticosteroids. Fatty cream base is an emollient and is therefore indicated in eczema. Podophyllum is used in warts, lidocaine is an anaesthetic, calcipotriol is used in psoriasis and clindamycin is used in acne.

A30   A

Amiodarone is an anti-arrhythmic drug indicated in supraventricular and ventricular arrhythmias. One of the main side-effects is photosensitivity and patients are advised to avoid exposure to sunlight and use sun protection factors.

A31   C

Rhinorrhoea and sneezing are characteristic symptoms of allergic rhinitis (hay fever). Fever and chesty cough indicate an upper respiratory tract infection. Headache and malaise are accompanying symptoms of common colds. Headache may also develop in allergic rhinitis because of congested sinuses.

A32   C

Calamine lotion is a combination of calamine and zinc oxide. It is mildly astringent and imparts a soothing antipruritic effect. Calamine lotion is cheap and effective with few restrictions on its use.

A33   B

Sodium alginate forms a 'raft' on the stomach contents leading to a reduction in reflux. Aluminium is an insoluble salt that is used as an antacid with no particular advantage in reflux. Chloroform water is a traditional preparation to reduce colic. Sucrose and lactose are sugars with no effect on - gastro-oesophageal reflux disease.

A34   C

Theophylline is a narrow therapeutic index drug with significant difference in bioavailability following oral administration. The half-life of the drug is increased by heart failure, cirrhosis and viral infections, in elderly patients, and by certain drugs, such as cimetidine, ciprofloxacin, oral contraceptives and fluvoxamine. The half-life is decreased in smokers, chronic alcoholism, and by certain drugs, such as phenytoin, rifampicin and carbamazepine.

A35   B

Itraconazole is a triazole antifungal causing side-effects, such as nausea, abdominal pain, dizziness and headache. Itraconazole does not lead to palpitations; however, it may lead to heart failure and hence itraconazole is administered with caution to patients at risk of heart failure.

A36   A

Dextromethorphan is an opioid antitussive similar in action to codeine and pholcodine. Codeine and pholcodine are considered to be more potent than dextromethorphan. Dextromethorphan tends to cause less constipation and dependence than codeine. Cough suppressants are not usually recommended in children under 2 years.

A37   A

Topical products for removal of corns and calluses often contain salicylic acid at a concentration of between 11% and 50% as a keratolytic agent in combination with lactic acid, the latter intended to aid absorption.

A38   D

Selenium sulphide, coal tar, ketoconazole and salicylic acid are agents that can be used in dandruff. Permethrin is an insecticide indicated in the eradication of head lice. Permethrin is available as alcoholic or aqueous lotions.

A39   D

Diverticulitis refers to the extension of mucosal pouches outwards from the external muscle wall into the gastrointestinal tract. Diverticulitis is accompanied by colicky pain lasting for a few days. The condition may be accompanied by constipation or diarrhoea and blood in stools.

A40   B

Raised intracranial pressure could be a cause of early morning headache. Early morning headache could also be triggered by sinusitis, tension or muscle spasm.

A41   C

Pregnancy is a common cause of early morning vomiting. The condition is referred to as morning sickness and may be relieved by taking dry biscuits on waking up.

A42   A

Tyrosine is the amino acid precursor of the sympathetic neurotransmitter noradrenaline.

A43   D

Tryptophan is the amino acid precursor of the neurotransmitter serotonin.

A44   C

Histidine is the amino acid precursor of the neurotransmitter histamine.

A45 C

Vitamin B$_2$ is another name for riboflavin.

A46 B

In osteoporosis calcium may be used in patients who are receiving bisphosphonates. Proprietary combination products such as Didronel PMO (disodium etidronate with calcium carbonate) are available.

A47 A

Folic acid is used as an adjunct to methotrexate therapy to limit methotrexate-induced side-effects such as mucositis and stomatitis.

A48 E

Retinol is contraindicated for use in pregnancy because of its teratogenic effect.

A49 A

Piperacillin is classified as a ureidopenicillin. It is active against *Pseudomonas aeruginosa.*

A50 C

Penicillin G, also referred to as benzylpenicillin, is inactivated by gastric acid and is therefore available only for injection.

A51 E

Flucloxacillin is an oral beta-lactam penicillin, which is resistant to the enzyme beta-lactamase and is therefore indicated in infections caused by penicillin-resistant organisms.

A52 C

Treatment of Crohn's disease is based on the administration of oral corticosteroids, to attain remission. Oral aminosalicylates, such as oral sulfasalazine, are indicated for long-term use as maintenance treatment. Oral corticosteroids are not indicated for maintenance treatment because of their side-effects.

A53   B

Patients with hyperthyroidism tend to have enhanced metabolism leading to weight loss, tremor and palpitations. Propranolol may be indicated to reduce the sympathetic symptoms, such as tremor and palpitations.

A54   E

Advanced age is a common predisposing factor to the development of osteoporosis.

A55   C

Topical application of corticosteroids may lead to spreading of local skin infections, striae and thinning of the skin. Topical preparations containing corticosteroids should not normally be applied for more than 7 days.

A56   C

Fibrinolytic agents, such as alteplase and urokinase, activate plasminogen to plasmin, which in turn degrades fibrin thereby breaking the thrombus and acting as thrombolytics. Fibrinolytic agents are indicated in acute myocardial infarction, venous thrombosis and embolism. Tranexamic acid is an antifibrinolytic agent consequently inhibiting fibrinolysis and bleeding.

A57   C

Ergotamine is an ergot derivative indicated for the treatment of migraine. Amitriptyline and propranolol can be used for the prophylaxis of migraine.

A58   A

All benzodiazepines are indicated in obsessive compulsive disorders. Diazepam and lorazepam are effective in status epilepticus, whereas chlordiazepoxide is indicated in alcohol withdrawal.

A59   B

Bromocriptine is a dopamine agonist acting by direct stimulation of the dopamine receptors. In Parkinson's disease, it is reserved for use in patients who are intolerant to levodopa or in whom levodopa alone is not sufficient. Orphenadrine is an antimuscarinic indicated in Parkinson's disease. Antimuscarinics tend to be more effective than levodopa in targeting tremor rather than rigidity and bradykinesia. Moclobemide is an antidepressant referred to as a reversible monoamine oxidase inhibitor (RIMA) type A.

A60   A

Doxycyline is a tetracycline antibiotic. All tetracylines are bacteriostatic, have a broad spectrum and are the treatment of choice for infections caused by *Chlamydia* and *Rickettsia* and in brucellosis. Doxycyline and minocyline are the only two tetracyclines that may be administered in renal impairment.

A61   B

Prescribers are expected to include the date of issue of the prescription and their signature.

A62   D

Tardive dyskinesia refers to uncontrollable facial movements. It is more likely to occur in the elderly. Tardive dyskinesia is commonly associated with the use of antipsychotic drugs, such as haloperidol. The atypical antipsychotics, such as clozapine, olanzapine, risperidone and quetiapine are less likely to cause tardive dyskinesia.

A63   B

Acute inflammation may be due to bacterial infection and trauma.

A64   E

Combined oral contraceptives are less likely to be associated with irregular vaginal bleeding than progestogen-only contraceptives. However, they are less suitable for smokers and breast-feeding women. They are more likely to cause deep-vein thrombosis than progestogen-only contraceptives.

A65   A

Conjunctivitis may be caused by viral infections, bacterial infections or infections caused by *Chlamydia*. Conjunctivitis caused by bacterial infections tends to be accompanied by a coloured discharge.

A66   E

Containers used for dispensing should always be labelled accordingly, preferably also with cautionary labels. Child-resistant containers may be difficult to use by elderly patients. Not all containers should be cleaned with alcohol before use as the medicine may interact with the alcohol.

A67   E

Clarithromycin is a macrolide that has a longer half-life than erythromycin so is administered twice daily. Clarithromycin is more active against Gram-positive organisms than erythromycin. Clarithromycin may be used in combination with amoxicillin, for example, as part of triple therapy used for the eradication of *Helicobacter pylori*.

A68   E

Asthma is managed by the use of an inhaled bronchodilator prescribed on an as-required (p.r.n.) basis to relieve acute attacks and administration of an inhaled corticosteroid as maintenance therapy. Budesonide is available as inhaled corticosteroid. Amoxicillin or another antibacterial agent may be required for short-term periods. Codeine, being an antitussive, should be used with caution in asthmatics and certainly not routinely.

A69   B

Side-effects and disadvantages of inhaled corticosteroids include hoarseness and oral candidiasis. Patients on inhaled corticosteroids are advised to rinse their mouth with water after using the inhaler, to reduce the occurrence of such side-effects. Adrenal suppression is a side-effect more likely to be associated with the long-term use of oral corticosteroids.

A70   C

Lactulose is an osmotic laxative acting by retaining fluid in the bowel. It takes a long time to act, generally up to 48 hours, and may cause abdominal discomfort.

A71   B

Hormone replacement therapy provides relief from vasomotor symptoms, decreases the risk of osteoporosis and decreases the risk of cardiovascular disease in post-menopausal women.

A72   D

Indometacin, which is a non-steroidal anti-inflammatory drug, inhibits the enzyme cyclo-oxygenase implicated in inflammatory reactions. Indometacin is more effective as an anti-inflammatory agent than ibuprofen and tends to have a higher side-effect profile, including headache, diarrhoea and gastro-intestinal disturbances. Rectal administration reduces but does not prevent gastrointestinal tract disturbances.

A73   D

Magnesium-containing antacids must be used with caution in renal impairment as the absorption of magnesium may lead to hypermagnesaemia with serious cardiovascular and neurological consequences. Magnesium-containing antacids tend to have a laxative effect and are often marketed in combination with aluminium-containing antacids to counteract the constipating effect of the aluminium antacid.

A74   B

Dexamethasone and betamethasone are corticosteroids available for topical application in eye products. Docusate sodium is indicated for ear wax removal.

A75   E

Referral for foot conditions is indicated in toenail involvement, diabetic patients and where foot colour and appearance are abnormal.

A76   E

When a drug is administered orally, the plasma drug concentration depends on the distribution pathways. For example, if the drug is present in high concentration in the hepatic portal vein, the occurrence of the first-pass effect decreases the amount of drug that reaches the circulation.

A77   A

Amenorrhoea, which refers to the absence of menstruation, is associated with anorexia nervosa, polycystic ovary syndrome and congenital adrenal hyperplasia. The condition requires referral.

A78   C

Antipsychotic drugs, such as flupentixol and haloperidol are the mainstay of treatment for acute attacks of mania. Lithium is not indicated as it may take a few days before the drug exerts an effect. Lithium may be given concomitantly with an antipsychotic drug.

A79   C

Back pain may be associated with osteoporosis and pregnancy. Osteomalacia refers to insufficient mineralisation of the bones, resulting in soft bones.

A80   B

Lorazepam is a short-acting benzodiazepine. Both short-acting and long-acting benzodiazepines, such as diazepam, may be indicated for short-term relief of severe anxiety.

A81 E

Sunscreen preparations tend to contain substances that protect the skin against sunburn caused by ultraviolet B (UVB) rays. UVA rays are associated with long-term skin damage. Sunscreen preparations contain a variety of sun protection factors but not necessarily a factor of 30.

A82 A

Carbocisteine is a mucolytic agent that may be used in chesty cough. Antihistamines tend to have antimuscarinic properties, resulting in urinary retention and are therefore contraindicated in prostatic hypertrophy.

A83 C

Eye drops should be discarded 4 weeks after opening because of loss of sterility of the product. Eye drops do contain preservatives.

A84 B

It is important to convey information about medications as directed according to the needs of each patient. Moreover the pharmacist must use appropriate, simple language and adjust according to the patient's age, personality and educational background.

A85 B

Methotrexate is an antimetabolite of folic acid and has immunosuppressant properties. It inhibits the enzyme dihydrofolate reductase that is required for the synthesis of purines and pyrimidines. It is used in malignant disease, Crohn's disease, rheumatic disease and psoriasis. Folic acid is given with methotrexate to reduce the occurrence of side-effects particularly the risk of mucositis.

A86 A

The occurrence of myocardial infarction is associated with onset of pain. One of the aims of treatment in the management of myocardial infarction is to pro-vide patient support and pain relief as soon as possible so as to reduce patient discomfort and anxiety. Intravenous administration of an opioid drug, usually diamorphine, is adopted and an anti-emetic drug is used to counteract the onset of nausea and vomiting.

A87 D

Morphine is an opioid analgesic that may be used for pain relief in myocardial infarction. However, diamorphine is usually preferred because it causes a lower risk of nausea and hypotension than morphine.

A88 B

Aspirin is acetylsalicylic acid and is used as an antiplatelet agent and for pain relief. Its use for anti-inflammatory effects is limited by the occurrence of side-effects, which include tinnitus and deafness, both features of salicylate poisoning.

A89 D

Indometacin is an indole acetic acid derivative, while naproxen is a propionic acid derivative. Both are non-steroidal anti-inflammatory drugs (NSAIDs). Indometacin is associated with a higher incidence of side-effects, particularly gastrointestinal as well as headache and dizziness.

A90 A

Mebendazole is a benzimidazole carbamate derivative that is used for the treatment of threadworm, roundworm, whipworm and hookworm infections. It is not recommended for women who are pregnant and in children under 2 years because the manufacturer reports that toxicity in animal studies has been reported.

A91 C

Fluocinolone is a potent corticosteroid anti-inflammatory agent.

A92   E

Dermatitis is a common inflammatory condition, which may require the use of a potent topical corticosteroid. Rosacea is a skin disorder whereby the blood vessels of the face become more prominent giving the face a flushed appearance. Urticaria refers to the appearance of red wheals, which may be due to an allergy.

A93   C

Carbimazole tends to cause neutropenia and patients are advised to report any sore throat to the pharmacist for referral. Blood counts would be required. Dry eyes are a consequence of hyperthyroidism and hypromellose eye drops could be recommended as a relief preparation.

A94   A

Cefuroxime is a second-generation cephalosporin with enhanced activity against *Haemophilus influenzae*, a Gram-negative organism. Side-effects include nausea, vomiting and headache.

A95   D

The patient should be advised to take cefuroxime tablets twice daily for 5 days. The patient should continue the carbimazole treatment. The patient should be advised to return to the pharmacist or to the physician if symptoms are aggravated during the cefuroxime treatment or if symptoms persist after the 5 days' antibacterial treatment.

A96–100

Cilest is a combined hormonal contraceptive that contains ethinylestradiol and norgestimate. These products may cause nausea, especially on commencement of therapy. Other side-effects that may occur in decreasing order of probability include fluid retention, reduced menstrual loss and photosensitivity. Acne is not commonly associated with combined hormonal contraceptive. Hormone therapy consisting of ethinylestradiol and cyproterone may be used for the management acne in women.

A96   5

A97   2

A98   1

A99   3

A100   4

Test 7

Questions

Questions 1–37

Directions: Each of the questions or incomplete statements is followed by five suggested answers. Select the best answer in each case.

Q1 The concentration of a solution of 120 mg of sodium hydroxide in 250 mL water expressed as %w/v is:

    A   ❑ 0.000 2
    B   ❑ 0.02
    C   ❑ 0.05
    D   ❑ 0.5
    E   ❑ 5

Q2 When advising a patient on the correct use of eye drops, which one of the following statements is *incorrect*?

    A   ❑ tilt your head back and pull down the lower lid of your eye with the index finger
    B   ❑ hold the tip of the dropper against the lower lid
    C   ❑ gently squeeze the dropper so that the correct number of drops are released
    D   ❑ close the eye for 2–3 minutes and wipe any excess liquid from your face with a tissue
    E   ❑ replace and tighten cap

Q3 Topical products for acne may contain benzoyl peroxide as a (an):

    A   ❑ antimicrobial
    B   ❑ emollient
    C   ❑ keratolytic
    D   ❑ bactericidal
    E   ❑ retinoid

Q4 Naproxen is classified as:

A ❑ a sulphonamide
B ❑ a corticosteroid
C ❑ a propionic acid derivative
D ❑ an anthraquinone
E ❑ an econazole

Q5 5000 mg equals 0.005:

A ❑ grams
B ❑ kilograms
C ❑ micrograms
D ❑ centigrams
E ❑ nanograms

Q6 Calculate the dose of a drug to be administered to a patient if the dosing regimen is listed as 5 mg/kg per day in divided doses every 8 hours. The patient weighs 67 kg:

A ❑ 67 mg t.d.s.
B ❑ 42 mg t.d.s.
C ❑ 335 mg t.d.s.
D ❑ 14 mg t.d.s.
E ❑ 112 mg t.d.s.

Q7 A pharmacist is required to dispense 30 g of 0.5% hydrocortisone ointment. The pharmacist has available a hydrocortisone ointment 1%. How many grams of the 1% ointment could be diluted with white soft paraffin to prepare this order?

A ❑ 15 g
B ❑ 30 g
C ❑ 0.15 g
D ❑ 0.5 g
E ❑ 1.5 g

Q8   Which one of the following agents is indicated for use as an anti-emetic agent?

A   ❑ docusate sodium
B   ❑ lansoprazole
C   ❑ ondansetron
D   ❑ ranitidine
E   ❑ mebeverine

Q9   The product that may be recommended safely for use by an infant with nasal congestion is:

A   ❑ topical pseudoephedrine
B   ❑ normal saline
C   ❑ systemic pseudoephedrine
D   ❑ cetirizine
E   ❑ mefenamic acid

Q10   A major target organ for gentamicin toxicity is the:

A   ❑ heart
B   ❑ liver
C   ❑ kidney
D   ❑ stomach
E   ❑ brain

Q11   Common side-effects of salbutamol include all EXCEPT:

A   ❑ fine tremor
B   ❑ tachycardia
C   ❑ headache
D   ❑ constipation
E   ❑ muscle cramps

Q12 Bezafibrate is a (an):

A ❏ lipid-regulating drug
B ❏ antihypertensive
C ❏ laxative
D ❏ antispasmodic
E ❏ calcium-channel blocker

Q13 What is the maximum adult daily dose for xylometazoline drops?

A ❏ three drops into each nostril three times daily
B ❏ one drop into each nostril three times daily
C ❏ three drops into each nostril six times daily
D ❏ one drop into each nostril twice daily
E ❏ six drops into each nostril three times daily

Q14 Citalopram is a (an):

A ❏ SSRI
B ❏ TCA
C ❏ antipsychotic
D ❏ benzodiazepine
E ❏ MAOI

Q15 The amount of diclofenac that is being administered per tablet of Voltarol tablets containing 25 mg diclofenac sodium is: (Diclofenac sodium has a molecular formula of $C_{14}H_{10}Cl_2NO_2.Na$; relative atomic mass of carbon = 12.01; hydrogen = 1.008; chlorine = 35.45; nitrogen = 14.01; sodium = 22.99; and oxygen = 16.00.)

A ❏ 20.99
B ❏ 21.98
C ❏ 23.19
D ❏ 24.27
E ❏ 25

Q16   The amount of morphine sulphate in milligrams that dissolves in 10 mL is (solubility 1 in 21):

A   ❑ 0.476
B   ❑ 2.1
C   ❑ 47.6
D   ❑ 476
E   ❑ 2100

Q17   What is the recommended dose of paracetamol for a child aged 5 years?

A   ❑ 250 mg every 4–6 hours
B   ❑ 125 mg every 4–6 hours
C   ❑ 500 mg every 4–6 hours
D   ❑ 250 mg every 6–8 hours
E   ❑ 125 mg every 6–8 hours

Q18   Levonorgestrel is a (an):

A   ❑ progestogen
B   ❑ oestrogen
C   ❑ prostaglandin
D   ❑ gonadorelin analogue
E   ❑ glucocorticoid

Q19   Aciclovir is indicated for the treatment of:

A   ❑ cold sores
B   ❑ erythema
C   ❑ measles
D   ❑ rubella
E   ❑ pruritus

Q20 Carbimazole is used in the treatment of:

A ❏ diabetes mellitus
B ❏ hyperthyroidism
C ❏ hypothyroidism
D ❏ carcinoma
E ❏ ulcerative colitis

Q21 Which one of the following antihistamines is least likely to cause sedation?

A ❏ diphenhydramine
B ❏ desloratadine
C ❏ chlorphenamine
D ❏ promethazine
E ❏ alimemazine

Q22 Alginic acid is found in some antacid preparations. The primary function is to:

A ❏ act as an antifoaming agent
B ❏ accelerate gastric emptying
C ❏ prevent refluxing into the oesophagus
D ❏ act as an antimuscarinic
E ❏ act as a flavouring agent

Q23 The use of a suspension as a parenteral preparation is contraindicated when the route of administration is:

A ❏ subcutaneous
B ❏ intramuscular
C ❏ intravenous
D ❏ intradermal
E ❏ intra-articular

Q24   Preparations used for infant colic contain:

A   ❏ simeticone
B   ❏ metoclopramide
C   ❏ domperidone
D   ❏ lactulose
E   ❏ ranitidine

Q25   Which of the following antibacterial drugs is NOT available for oral administration?

A   ❏ tetracycline
B   ❏ fusidic acid
C   ❏ gentamicin
D   ❏ erythromycin
E   ❏ ciprofloxacin

Q26   All of the following are viral infections EXCEPT:

A   ❏ chickenpox
B   ❏ tinea pedis
C   ❏ hepatitis
D   ❏ mumps
E   ❏ rubella

Q27   A tourist comes to the pharmacy asking for a sun lotion for sun protection. Which product would you recommend?

A   ❏ tanning oil SPF 4
B   ❏ tanning oil SPF 8
C   ❏ lotion SPF 2
D   ❏ lotion SPF 6
E   ❏ lotion SPF 8

Q28   Bioavailability describes the relative amount of drug that reaches the:

A   ❑ kidney
B   ❑ systemic circulation
C   ❑ liver
D   ❑ stomach
E   ❑ small intestine

Q29   When a drug is administered as a solid oral dosage form, the first process that occurs is:

A   ❑ absorption
B   ❑ disintegration
C   ❑ dissolution
D   ❑ ionisation
E   ❑ metabolism

Q30   Which of the following agents is NOT employed in the treatment of depression?

A   ❑ lorazepam
B   ❑ imipramine
C   ❑ paroxetine
D   ❑ venlafaxine
E   ❑ moclobemide

Q31   For which of the following is immunisation NOT provided to children:

A   ❑ measles
B   ❑ mumps
C   ❑ infectious mononucleosis
D   ❑ rubella
E   ❑ diphtheria

Q32   Rubella virus has the most serious effect on:

A   ❏ a pregnant woman
B   ❏ an adolescent girl
C   ❏ a fetus
D   ❏ a diabetic patient
E   ❏ a newborn infant

Q33   The first-line of treatment of rheumathoid arthritis is:

A   ❏ sodium aurothiomalate
B   ❏ paracetamol
C   ❏ indometacin
D   ❏ diclofenac
E   ❏ dexamethasone

Q34   Which of the following drugs should be used with utmost caution in a patient who had a severe allergic reaction to penicillin?

A   ❏ clindamycin
B   ❏ ketoconazole
C   ❏ cefaclor
D   ❏ vancomycin
E   ❏ erythromycin

Q35   Which of the following non-steroidal anti-inflammatory drugs would be useful for short-term treatment in a patient with arthritis who also complains of dyspepsia from time to time?

A   ❏ diclofenac potassium
B   ❏ aspirin
C   ❏ indometacin
D   ❏ meloxicam
E   ❏ diclofenac sodium

Q36   Paracetamol overdose is most likely to cause:

   A   ❑ renal damage
   B   ❑ tinnitus
   C   ❑ hepatic necrosis
   D   ❑ seizures
   E   ❑ ataxia

Q37   The drug of choice in prolonged febrile convulsions is:

   A   ❑ carbamazepine
   B   ❑ diazepam
   C   ❑ phenytoin
   D   ❑ paracetamol
   E   ❑ mefenamic acid

Questions 38–61

Directions: Each group of questions below consists of five lettered headings followed by a list of numbered questions. For each numbered question select the one heading that is most closely related to it. Each heading may be used once, more than once, or not at all.

Questions 38–40 concern the following corticosteroids:

   A   ❑ hydrocortisone
   B   ❑ hydrocortisone butyrate
   C   ❑ fluocinolone
   D   ❑ fluticasone
   E   ❑ clobetasone

Select, from A to E, which one of the above:

Q38   is available orally

Q39   is the least potent

Q40   is available for inhalation

Questions 41–43 concern the following diuretics:

A   ❑ furosemide
B   ❑ bendroflumethiazide
C   ❑ spironolactone
D   ❑ metolazone
E   ❑ indapamide

Select, from A to E, which one of the above:

Q41   inhibits re-absorption from ascending loop of Henle in renal tubule

Q42   should be used with caution in patients with enlarged prostate

Q43   is a potassium-sparing diuretic

Questions 44–47 concern the following antipsychotic drugs:

A   ❑ chlorpromazine
B   ❑ flupentixol
C   ❑ haloperidol
D   ❑ clozapine
E   ❑ prochlorperazine

Select, from A to E, which one of the above:

Q44   is associated with pronounced sedative effects

Q45   is indicated in agitation and restlessness in the elderly, despite the high incidence of extrapyramidal side-effects

Q46   is classified as a thioxanthene antipsychotic drug

Q47   may be associated with the occurrence of hyperglycaemia and diabetes

Questions 48–50 concern the following drugs:

A   ❑ benzocaine
B   ❑ irinotecan
C   ❑ galantamine
D   ❑ paclitaxel
E   ❑ simvastatin

Select, from A to E, which one of the above:

Q48   was synthesised to mimic the nerve-blocking activity of cocaine

Q49   is indicated for dementia in Alzheimer's disease

Q50   was originally derived from the bark of the yew tree

Questions 51–54 concern the following drugs:

A   ❑ clarithromycin
B   ❑ glyceryl trinitrate
C   ❑ imipramine
D   ❑ sumatriptan
E   ❑ valsartan

Select, from A to E, which one of the above results in a clinically significant interaction with:

Q51   alcohol

Q52   potassium salts

Q53   tramadol

Q54   simvastatin

Questions 55–58: Match the lettered dosage strength with its most closely corresponding numbered generic name

A   ❏ 20 mg
B   ❏ 500 mg
C   ❏ 5 mg
D   ❏ 100 mg
E   ❏ 75 mg

Select, from A to E, which one of the above dosages is used for:

Q55   atenolol tablets

Q56   prednisolone tablets

Q57   ranitidine tablets

Q58   paracetamol tablets

Questions 59–61 concern the following preparations:

A ❏ ascorbic acid
B ❏ acetylsalicylic acid
C ❏ thiamine
D ❏ acetaminophen
E ❏ fluoride

Select, from A to E, which one of the above is the chemical name for:

Q59 aspirin

Q60 paracetamol

Q61 vitamin C

Questions 62–78

Directions: For each of the questions below, ONE or MORE of the responses is (are) correct. Decide which of the responses is (are) correct. Then choose:

A ❏ if 1, 2 and 3 are correct
B ❏ if 1 and 2 only are correct
C ❏ if 2 and 3 only are correct
D ❏ if 1 only is correct
E ❏ if 3 only is correct

Directions summarised				
A	**B**	**C**	**D**	**E**
1, 2, 3	1, 2 only	2, 3 only	1 only	3 only

Q62   A patient with hypertension should be advised to avoid:

1   ❏ antihistamines
2   ❏ oral rehydration salts
3   ❏ sympathomimetics

Q63   Naproxen:

1   ❏ inhibits prostaglandin synthesis
2   ❏ inhibits bradykinin release
3   ❏ increases body temperature

Q64   In pharmaceutical manufacturing, process validation:

1   ❏ is a GMP requirement
2   ❏ aims to ensure that the final product produced is of the expected quality
3   ❏ should be carried out independently by the quality assurance department

Q65   Angiotensin-converting enzyme inhibitors should be used with caution in patients:

1   ❏ receiving diuretics
2   ❏ with renal disease
3   ❏ with hypertension

Q66   When dispensing sublingual glyceryl trinitrate tablets to a patient, they should be advised to:

1   ❏ discard tablets 8 weeks after opening
2   ❏ keep tablets in original container and keep tightly closed
3   ❏ chew tablets as necessary

Q67   The following drugs may precipitate an asthma attack:

1   ❏ beta-adrenoceptor blockers
2   ❏ non-steroidal anti-inflammatory drugs
3   ❏ paracetamol

Q68 Which of the following agents is (are) indicated for the prophylaxis of migraine headache?

1 ❑ ergotamine
2 ❑ propranolol
3 ❑ amitriptyline

Q69 Medicines associated with anaphylactic shock include:

1 ❑ antibacterial agents
2 ❑ vaccines
3 ❑ NSAIDS

Q70 Ipratropium bromide:

1 ❑ is an antimuscarinic agent
2 ❑ is contraindicated in asthma patients
3 ❑ is only available as a solid oral dosage form

Q71 Acetazolamide:

1 ❑ may be used in the treatment of glaucoma
2 ❑ is a carbonic anhydrase inhibitor
3 ❑ is available as eye drops

Q72 Warfarin:

1 ❑ is available as 1, 3, 5 mg tablets
2 ❑ has hypersensitivity as the main adverse effect
3 ❑ price per tablet is about €2.5 (£1.60)

Q73 Chlorhexidine gluconate:

1 ❑ inhibits the formation of plaque on teeth
2 ❑ when used as a mouthwash may cause teeth staining
3 ❑ has antiseptic properties

Q74   Antibacterial agents used topically in the treatment of acne include:

1   ❏ erythromycin
2   ❏ tetracycline
3   ❏ isotretinoin

Q75   Acid rebound is likely to occur with the chronic use of large doses of which of the following preparations?

1   ❏ aluminium hydroxide
2   ❏ magnesium hydroxide
3   ❏ calcium carbonate

Q76   Which of the following drugs would be effective in the treatment of Parkinson's disease?

1   ❏ co-careldopa
2   ❏ orphenadrine
3   ❏ trifluoperazine

Q77   Metronidazole:

1   ❏ is an antifungal agent
2   ❏ is active against protozoa
3   ❏ causes disulfiram-like reaction with alcohol

Q78   For the treatment of corns and calluses:

1   ❏ salicylic acid is used as a keratolytic
2   ❏ epidermabrasion is a safe method of treatment
3   ❏ imidazole antifungals may be recommended

Questions 79–82

Directions: The following questions consist of a first statement
followed by a second statement. Decide whether the first
statement is true or false. Decide whether the second
statement is true or false. Then choose:

A   ❑ if both statements are true and the second statement is a *cor-rect explanation* of the first statement

B   ❑ if both statements are true but the second statement *is NOT a correct explanation* of the first statement

C   ❑ if the first statement is true but the second statement is false

D   ❑ if the first statement is false but the second statement is true

E   ❑ if both statements are false

Directions summarised		
	First statement	**Second statement**
A	True	True	Second statement is a *correct explanation* of the first
B	True	True	Second statement is *NOT a correct explanation* of the first
C	True	False	
D	False	True	
E	False	False	

Q79   Loperamide can be used in children over 3 months. Loperamide is an adsorbent drug.

Q80   Tardive dyskinesia is a chronic movement disorder characterised by uncontrolled facial movements. Tardive dyskinesia is associated with the use of trifluoperazine.

Q81   Beclometasone aerosol is used in the acute asthmatic attack. When used in conjunction with a bronchodilator administered by inhalation, the bronchodilator should be used first.

Q82   Diuretic therapy is interrupted for 1 month when ACE inhibitors are being added to a patient's drug therapy. Diuretics interfere with the action of ACE inhibitors.

Questions 83–100

Directions: These questions involve cases. Read the prescription or case and answer the questions.

Questions 83–87: Use the prescription below

Patient's name: . . . .
Age: 34 years Clarithromycin 250 mg tablets b.d.   m. 10 Codeine linctus 10 mL b.d.   m. 1 bottle . . . .
Doctor's signature: . . . .

Q83   Codeine linctus:

1   ❑ may be useful if sleep is disturbed by coughing
2   ❑ improves sputum expectoration
3   ❑ is useful when the cough is occurring as a side-effect of another drug

A   ❑ 1, 2, 3
B   ❑ 1, 2 only
C   ❑ 2, 3 only
D   ❑ 1 only
E   ❑ 3 only

Q84   Clarithromycin:

1   ❑ is a derivative of neomycin
2   ❑ dosage frequency may be increased to three times daily
3   ❑ should be used with caution in patients who are predisposed to QT interval prolongation

A   ❑ 1, 2, 3
B   ❑ 1, 2 only
C   ❑ 2, 3 only
D   ❑ 1 only
E   ❑ 3 only

Q85   The patient develops vaginal thrush superinfection. The most appropriate treatment is:

A   ❑ povidone-iodine
B   ❑ clindamycin
C   ❑ econazole
D   ❑ sulphonamide
E   ❑ penicillins

Q86   Which of the following have to be avoided when the patient is taking clarithromycin?

A   ❏ bumetanide
B   ❏ warfarin
C   ❏ cimetidine
D   ❏ naproxen
E   ❏ phenylephrine

Q87   Which of the following auxiliary labels should be used during dispensing?

1   ❏ 'May cause drowsiness. If affected do not drive or operate machinery'
2   ❏ 'Take at regular intervals. Complete the prescribed course unless otherwise directed'
3   ❏ 'Avoid exposure of skin to direct sunlight or sunlamps'

A   ❏ 1, 2, 3
B   ❏ 1, 2 only
C   ❏ 2, 3 only
D   ❏ 1 only
E   ❏ 3 only

Questions 88–91: Use the prescription below

Patient's name: . . . .

Age: 45 years
conjugated oestrogen 625 µg/norgestrel 150 µg tablets
1 daily   repeat for 3 months

Doctor's signature: . . . .

Q88   Risks associated with the use of this combination product include:

1   ❑ stroke
2   ❑ ovarian cancer
3   ❑ osteoporosis

A   ❑ 1, 2, 3
B   ❑ 1, 2 only
C   ❑ 2, 3 only
D   ❑ 1 only
E   ❑ 3 only

Q89   The patient is advised to:

1   ❑ have a 7-day interval between the three courses
2   ❑ take one tablet daily
3   ❑ start subsequent courses without interval

A   ❑ 1, 2, 3
B   ❑ 1, 2 only
C   ❑ 2, 3 only
D   ❑ 1 only
E   ❑ 3 only

Q90   Absolute contraindications to the use of this combination product are:

1   ❑ thromboembolic disorders
2   ❑ oestrogen-dependent carcinoma
3   ❑ history of migraine

A   ❑ 1, 2, 3
B   ❑ 1, 2 only
C   ❑ 2, 3 only
D   ❑ 1 only
E   ❑ 3 only

Q91   Other dosage forms available for the same line of treatment include:

1   ❏ self-adhesive patches
2   ❏ cream
3   ❏ pessaries

A   ❏ 1, 2, 3
B   ❏ 1, 2 only
C   ❏ 2, 3 only
D   ❏ 1 only
E   ❏ 3 only

Questions 92–94: Use the case below:

A 24-year-old woman comes to the pharmacy with a new prescription for amitriptyline 25 mg tablets, two tablets t.d.s.

Q92   When dispensing the above prescription the pharmacist should advise the patient that side-effects to be expected are:

1   ❏ increased micturition
2   ❏ heartburn
3   ❏ drowsiness

A   ❏ 1, 2, 3
B   ❏ 1, 2 only
C   ❏ 2, 3 only
D   ❏ 1 only
E   ❏ 3 only

Q93   The label produced for the medicine dispensed to the patient should include:

A   ❏ take two tablets three times daily
B   ❏ take two tablets four times daily
C   ❏ take two tablets three times daily after meals
D   ❏ take two tablets three times daily before meals
E   ❏ take one tablet three times daily

Q94 The patient returns to the pharmacy after 4 days complaining that the drug is causing dry mouth, constipation and that the drug has not improved the symptoms of depression. The pharmacist should:

A ❏ tell the patient to stop taking the medication

B ❏ explain to the patient that these are expected side-effects of early treatment of the drug

C ❏ contact the prescriber that the drug is not effective in this patient

D ❏ contact the prescriber and report that the patient is suffering a hypersensitivity reaction to the drug

E ❏ inform the prescriber that an anticholinergic agent needs to be prescribed to this patient

Questions 95–96: Use the prescription below

Patient's name: . . . .

Age: 21 years
clindamycin capsules 75 mg
b.d. m. 180

Doctor's signature: . . . .

Q95 The patient states that they were prescribed for acne. The treatment duration is:

A ❏ at least 3 months

B ❏ not exceeding 3 days

C ❏ 5 days

D ❏ 2 weeks

E ❏ not exceeding 4 weeks

Q96   Clindamycin:

1   ❏ is a penicillin
2   ❏ is a broad-spectrum antibacterial agent
3   ❏ may cause antibiotic-associated colitis

A   ❏ 1, 2, 3
B   ❏ 1, 2 only
C   ❏ 2, 3 only
D   ❏ 1 only
E   ❏ 3 only

Questions 97–100: Use the prescription below

```
Patient's name:         . . . . . . . . . . . . . . . . . . . . . . .

Age: 68 years
glibenclamide 5 mg tablets
o.m. m. 30




Doctor's signature:     . . . . . . . . . . . . . . . . . . . . . . . .
```

Q97   Glibenclamide acts mainly by:

A   ❏ increasing insulin secretion
B   ❏ regulating carbohydrate metabolism
C   ❏ decreasing gluconeogenesis
D   ❏ increasing utilisation of glucose
E   ❏ delaying absorption of starch

Q98   Hypoglycaemia may develop if the patient:

1   ❏ skips meals
2   ❏ follows a weight-reducing diet
3   ❏ misses glibenclamide tablets

A   ❏ 1, 2, 3
B   ❏ 1, 2 only
C   ❏ 2, 3 only
D   ❏ 1 only
E   ❏ 3 only

Q99   Signs that indicate hypoglycaemia include:

1   ❏ nausea and vomiting
2   ❏ perspiration
3   ❏ palpitations

A   ❏ 1, 2, 3
B   ❏ 1, 2 only
C   ❏ 2, 3 only
D   ❏ 1 only
E   ❏ 3 only

Q100 The patient returns to the pharmacy complaining of very frequent attacks of hypoglycaemia, especially during the night. When contacted by the prescriber, which alternative treatment may be recommended?:

A   ❏ chlorpropamide
B   ❏ acarbose
C   ❏ gliclazide
D   ❏ repaglinide
E   ❏ insulin

Test 7

Answers

A1 C

The solution consists of 0.12 g (120 mg) in 250 mL which in %w/v is 0.05% (0.12 × 100/250).

A2 B

When dispensing eye drops, patients are advised to tilt back their head, pull down the lower eyelid with the index finger and instil the drops without touching the eyelid with tip of the dropper. Patients are then advised to keep their eyes closed for 2–3 minutes. Any excess liquid drops can be wiped away from the face. The eye dropper is replaced and capped. Patients applying more than one type of eye drops are advised to allow an interval of 5 minutes between one medication and another.

A3 C

Benzoyl peroxide promotes the shedding of keratinised epithelial cells on the skin and is therefore a keratolytic agent. In the treatment of acne it is indicated as a first-line agent in the form of topical preparations. Benzoyl peroxide is mildly irritant, particularly during the early stages of treatment and hence a low strength is chosen to initiate treatment. Moreover aqueous preparations are preferred over alcoholic preparations, to avoid irritation.

A4 C

Naproxen is a non-steroidal anti-inflammatory agent classified as a propionic acid derivative.

A5 B

An amount of 5000 mg is equivalent to 5 g, which is equivalent to 0.005 kg.

A6   E

The daily dose for a patient weighing 67 kg is 335 mg (67 × 5), meaning that the drug must be administered 112 mg three times daily (every 8 hours).

A7   A

Ointments are given as w/w%. Therefore 1% hydrocortisone ointment is equivalent to 1 g of hydrocortisone per 100 g of ointment.

Hence:

> 0.5 g hydrocortisone per 100 g ointment
> = ? g per 30 g
> = (30 g × 0.5)/100 g
> = 0.15 g hydrocortisone in 30 g ointment.
> 1 g hydrocortisone in 100 g ointment
> = 0.15 g in ? g hydrocortisone 1%
> = 100 g × 0.15 g
> = 15 g hydrocortisone 1%.

Therefore 15 g of the 1% hydrocortisone ointment need to be diluted with white soft paraffin to make up 30 g of 0.5% hydrocortisone ointment.

A8   C

Ondansetron is a $5HT_3$ antagonist indicated as an anti-emetic agent in nausea and vomiting associated with chemotherapy. The dose administered depends on the emetogenic degree of the chemotherapeutic agents used.

A9   B

Normal saline (0.9%) relieves nasal congestion by liquifying mucous secretions thereby acting as a nasal decongestant. It is safely recommended for use in infants. Topical administration of sympathomimetic nasal decongestants such as pseudoephedrine in infants may lead to irritation with narrowing of the nasal passages. Systemic use of the sympathomimetics increases the risk of side-effects, such as tachycardia, making systemic use of nasal decongestants all the more contraindicated in infants. Cetirizine is a non-sedating antihistamine. Antihistamines tend to be more effective in reducing rhinor-rhoea and sneezing rather than nasal congestion. Mefenamic acid is a non-steroidal anti-inflammatory.

A10   C

Gentamicin is an aminoglycoside. All aminoglycosides tend to be nephrotoxic and ototoxic. The dose must be reduced and serum concentrations must be monitored in patients with impaired renal function. Concomitant administra-tion of aminoglycosides and other nephrotoxic drugs, such as certain diuretics, ciclosporin, teicoplanin and vancomycin should be avoided.

A11   D

Salbutamol is a selective $beta_2$-agonist and therefore mimics the sympathetic system resulting in tachycardia and fine tremor. Salbutamol causes potassium loss leading to the development of muscle cramps. It also leads to headache. Constipation is not a side-effect of salbutamol but is commonly associated with the use of antimuscarinics.

A12   A

Bezafibrate is a lipid-regulating drug classified as a fibrate. Fibrates act by reducing the serum triglycerides and low-density lipoproteins (LDLs) and rais-ing high-density lipoprotein (HDL) cholesterol levels. Statins, which inhibit the enzyme 3-hydroxy-3-methylglutaryl coenzyme A (HMG CoA), tend to be less effective than fibrates in reducing triglyceride levels and raising the HDL cho-lesterol levels but more effective than the fibrates in lowering LDL cholesterol levels.

A13   A

Xylometazoline is a nasal decongestant. The maximum adult dose recom-mended is two drops into each nostril three times daily. The drops are not rec-ommended for children under 2 years of age.

A14   A

Citalopram is a selective serotonin re-uptake inhibitor (SSRI). These tend to have fewer antimuscarinic effects than tricyclic antidepressant (TCA) drugs, such as dry mouth and constipation; however, SSRIs tend to cause gastro-intestinal effects, such as nausea and vomiting. MAOIs are monoamine oxidase inhibitors.

A15   C

1 mole diclofenac weighs: $(12.01 \times 4) + (1.008 \times 10) + (35.45 \times 2) + 14.01 + (16.00 \times 2) = 295.13$ g; 1 mole diclofenac sodium weighs $295.13 + 22.99 = 318.12$ g. Diclofenac: diclofenac sodium as 295.13: 318.12 and therefore 23.19 mg ($295.13 \times 25/318.12$): 25 mg.

A16   D

In 21 mL, 1 g morphine sulphate is dissolved. In 10 mL, 0.476 g (10/21) or 476 mg can be dissolved.

A17   A

The recommended dose of paracetamol for a 5-year-old child is 250 mg every 4–6 hours up to a maximum of 4 doses in 24 hours.

A18   A

Levonorgestrel is a progestogen derivative. It is found either in combined oral contraceptives coupled with an oestrogen derivative or alone in progestogen-only contraceptives.

A19   A

Aciclovir is an antiviral indicated in the treatment and prophylaxis of cold sores. It is available for systemic administration (tablets) or topical use (cream, eye ointment). In the management of cold sores, the cream is applied every 4 hours and continued for 5 days. Its use should be started as soon as symptoms (tingling sensation) begin.

A20 B

Carbimazole is an antithyroid drug indicated in hyperthyroidism. It is usually administered as 15 mg daily in the morning. Carbimazole tends to cause agranulocytosis and therefore patients are advised to report immediately any signs of infections, such as sore throat.

A21 B

Desloratadine is a non-sedating antihistamine. Diphenhydramine, chlorphenamine, promethazine and alimemazine are sedating antihistamines with diphenhydramine and promethazine being marketed in over-the-counter hypnotic preparations.

A22 C

Alginic acid tends to prevent gastro-oesophageal reflux. The antifoaming agent intended to relieve flatulence is simeticone.

A23 C

Parenteral preparations in the form of a suspension cannot be administered through the intravenous route. Preparations intended for administration in this way must be soluble solutions to avoid occlusion of the veins.

A24 A

Simeticone is an antifoaming agent that relieves flatulence and is used in infant colic.

A25 C

Gentamicin is an aminoglycoside. As aminoglycosides are not absorbed from the gastrointestinal tract, gentamicin is only presented for parenteral or topical use (as eye/ear drops).

A26   B

Tinea pedis is a fungal infection commonly known as athlete's foot. Chickenpox is a childhood infection caused by the herpes zoster virus. Hepatitis is a viral infection of the liver. Mumps is a viral infection characterised by bilateral or unilateral inflammation of the salivary glands. Rubella (German measles) is caused by the rubella virus.

A27   E

Sunscreen preparations with a sun protection factor of eight allow people to stay in the sun without burning eight times longer than those not using any sun protection factor. The higher the factor the greater the degree of protection.

A28   B

Bioavailability is defined as the relative amount of drug that reaches the systemic circulation and the rate at which the drug appears in the circulation.

A29   B

Disintegration into fine particles is the first process that occurs when a drug is administered as a solid oral dosage form. The effectiveness of a tablet or solid dosage form in releasing the drug depends on the rate of disintegration. Dissolution rate is the rate at which the solid fine particles dissolve in a solvent.

A30   A

Lorazepam is a short-acting benzodiazepine indicated for use in relieving anxiety and insomnia. Lorazepam may also be administered perioperatively to alleviate pain and in status epilepticus. Imipramine is a tricyclic antidepressant, paroxetine is a selective serotonin re-uptake inhibitor, venlafaxine is a serotonin and adrenaline re-uptake inhibitor and moclobemide is a reversible monoamine oxidase inhibitor. Imipramine, paroxetine, venlafaxine and moclobemide are all classified as antidepressants.

A31 C

Common childhood vaccines include the three-in-one measles, mumps and rubella and the diphtheria vaccine. Infectious mononucleosis, also known as glandular fever, is caused by the Epstein-Barr virus and no vaccine is available.

A32 C

The rubella virus results in a self-limiting infection characterised by a rash spreading from the face, trunk and limbs. The infection commonly occurs in children. The rubella virus has the most serious effect on the fetus. Rubella occurring during pregnancy, especially during the first trimester, may result in spontaneous abortion, stillbirths or congenital malformations.

A33 D

The first-line agents in the treatment of rheumatoid arthritis are non-steroidal anti-inflammatory drugs such as diclofenac. Diclofenac and indometacin, another NSAID, tend to have similar activity; however, indometacin has a higher incidence of side-effects and therefore diclofenac is more appropriate for initial treatment. Sodium aurothiomalate is classified as a disease-modifying antirheumatic drug and is used as a second-line treatment in rheumatoid arthritis, but has been superseded by methotrexate, administered weekly. Paracetamol is often indicated in the management of osteoarthritis. Local intra-articular injections of dexamethasone may be administered for the relief of soft-tissue inflammatory conditions.

A34 C

Patients allergic to penicillin may be cross-sensitive to cephalosporins. Cephalosporins (cefaclor, first-generation cephalosporin) are therefore avoided in these patients and instead macrolides (for example, erythromycin) are generally administered. Ketoconazole is an imidazole antifungal agent.

A35   D

Meloxicam is a partially selective cyclo-oxygenase-2 inhibitor and is therefore less likely to cause gastrointestinal side-effects, such as bleeding, than other NSAIDs.

A36   C

Paracetamol overdose is most likely to cause hepatic necrosis and to a lesser extent renal necrosis. Hepatic necrosis is maximal within 3–4 hours of ingestion and may lead to encephalopathy, haemorrhage, hypoglycaemia, cerebral oedema and death. Acetylcysteine tends to protect the liver if given within 10–12 hours of paracetamol poisoning. The maximum adult dose of paracetamol is 4 g in 24 hours.

A37   B

Diazepam, a long-acting benzodiazepine can be used either intravenously (risk of thrombophlebitis) or intramuscularly or rectally (both of the last two routes are associated with slow absorption).

A38   A

Hydrocortisone is available orally. Other corticosteroids also available orally include prednisolone, betamethasone, cortisone acetate, methylprednisolone, dexamethasone and fluocortolone.

A39   A

Hydrocortisone is the least potent corticosteroid.

A40   D

Fluticasone is available for inhalation as Flixotide inhaler as well as Flixonase nasal spray.

A41   A

Furosemide, a loop diuretic, inhibits re-absorption from the ascending loop of Henle in the renal tubule.

A42   A

Loop diuretics should be used with caution in patients with urinary retention, for example, patients with enlarged prostate as they may cause urinary retention. Small doses and less potent diuretics should be used.

A43   C

Spironolactone is a potassium-sparing diuretic. It is an aldosterone antagonist and potentiates the action of loop or thiazide diuretics.

A44   A

Chlorpromazine is an aliphatic antipsychotic with marked sedative properties.

A45   C

Haloperidol is a butyrophenone that is associated with a high incidence of extrapyramidal side-effects. It brings about a rapid control of agitation and restlessness and is preferred to chlorpromazine in the elderly because it causes less hypotension.

A46   B

Flupentixol is an antipsychotic classified as a thioxanthene. Thioxanthenes have pronounced extrapyramidal side-effects.

A47   D

Clozapine is an atypical antipsychotic that is usually used in patients who are inadequately controlled with other antipsychotics. The reason is that clozapine is associated with a risk of potentially fatal agranulocytosis. As with other atypicals, side-effects of clozapine include occurrence of hyperglycaemia and diabetes.

A48   A

Benzocaine is an anaesthetic drug that was originally synthesised to mimic the nerve blocking activity of cocaine.

A49   C

Galantamine is a reversible inhibitor of acetylcholinesterase that also possesses nicotinic receptor agonist properties, and which is used in mild-to-moderate dementia in Alzheimer's disease.

A50   D

Paclitaxel is a taxane that was originally derived from the bark of the yew tree. Paclitaxel is used in cytotoxic chemotherapy for malignant disease.

A51   C

Imipramine is a tricyclic antidepressant and when it is administered con-comitantly with alcohol, increased sedation occurs.

A52   E

Valsartan is an angiotensin-II receptor antagonist and when administered to patients receiving potassium salts, the risk of hyperkalaemia is increased.

A53   C

Tramadol is an opioid analgesic and when given to patients who are also receiving imipramine (a tricyclic antidepressant), there is an increased risk of central nervous system toxicity. The risk of occurrence of sedation is increased.

A54   A

Simvastastin is a statin and there is an increased risk of myopathy when simvastatin is given with clarithromycin (macrolide).

A55   D

Atenolol (water soluble beta-adrenoceptor blocker) is available as 25 mg, 50 mg or 100 mg tablets.

A56   C

Prednisolone (corticosteroid) is available as 1 mg, 2.5 mg, 5 mg and 25 mg tablets.

A57   E

Ranitidine (H$_2$-receptor antagonist) is available as 75 mg, 150 mg and 300 mg tablets.

A58   B

Paracetamol is available as 500 mg tablets.

A59   B

Acetylsalicylic acid is the chemical name for aspirin.

A60   D

Acetaminophen is the chemical name for paracetamol.

A61   A

Ascorbic acid is the chemical name for vitamin C.

A62   C

Sympathomimetics mimic the sympathetic system, thereby increasing the force of contraction of the heart and the blood pressure. Sympathomimetics are therefore contraindicated in patients with hypertension. Oral rehydration salts consist of electrolytes including sodium and therefore should be used with care. The advantages of oral rehydration salts in diarrhoea outweigh this disadvantage.

A63   D

Naproxen, a non-steroidal anti-inflammatory drug, inhibits prostaglandin release through inhibition of the cyclo-oxygenase-2 enzyme, producing an analgesic and anti-inflammatory effect.

A64   B

In pharmaceutical manufacturing, process validation is an exercise that requires the contribution from different departments, including quality assurance and quality control. It is a requirement for good manufacturing practice (GMP) to ensure that the final product produced is of the expected quality.

A65   B

Angiotensin-converting enzyme inhibitors should be used with caution in patients taking diuretics because of an enhanced hypotensive effect. Angiotensin-converting enzyme inhibitors should also be used with caution in patients with renal impairment. Renal function needs to be monitored in patients with renovascular disease.

A66   B

Patients using sublingual glyceryl trinitrate tablets are advised to take a tablet at the first sign of angina. Patients can take three sublingual tablets in 15 minutes after which they must seek professional advice. Patients are advised to keep the tablets handy and in the original container because of instability. The tablets should be dissolved sublingually and not chewed. The tablets must be discarded 8 weeks after opening.

A67   B

Beta-adrenoceptor blockers block the sympathetic system antagonising the effect on the lungs, resulting in bronchoconstriction. Non-steroidal anti-inflammatory drugs inhibit prostaglandin synthesis, which may lead to bronchoconstriction.

A68   C

Ergotamine is an ergot alkaloid derivative indicated in the treatment of migraine. Propranolol (a fat-soluble and therefore centrally active beta-blocker) and amitriptyline (tricyclic antidepressant) are used for the prophy-laxis of migraine headache.

A69   A

Antibacterial agents, vaccines and non-steroidal anti-inflammatory drugs (NSAIDs) may all lead to anaphylactic shock if the patient is allergic to these products.

A70   D

Ipratropium bromide is an antimuscarinic agent indicated in asthma and in chronic obstructive pulmonary disease but it is more effective in the latter. The drug is available only for inhalation because of the potential side-effects if given orally.

A71   B

Acetazolamide is a carbonic anhydrase inhibitor, which reduces intraocular pressure by reducing aqueous humour production. It is used in the treatment of glaucoma. Acetazolamide is administered systemically. Recently newer carbonic anhydrase inhibitors have been developed, which are available as topical agents (for example, dorzolamide).

A72   D

Warfarin is an oral anticoagulant agent available as 1 mg (brown tablets), 3 mg (blue tablets) and 5 mg (pink tablets). The main side-effect of warfarin is increased bleeding. The approximate price of warfarin per tablet is €0.014 (£0.013).

A73   A

Chlorhexidine gluconate inhibits the formation of plaque on teeth and is indicated in oral infections and periodontal disease. Long-term use of chlorhexidine mouthwash may result in staining of the teeth. Chlorhexidine has antiseptic properties.

A74 B

Antibacterial preparations that may be used topically in acne include erythromycin, tetracycline and clindamycin. Isotretinoin is a tretinoin isomer used in the management of acne.

A75 E

Antacids containing calcium carbonate have the greatest neutralising capacity but tend to cause acid rebound with long-term use. Calcium carbonate may also lead to hypercalcaemia and the milk-alkali syndrome, which is characterised by nausea, headache and renal damage.

A76 B

Co-careldopa is a combination of levodopa and the peripheral dopadecarboxylase inhibitor. Co-careldopa is indicated in Parkinson's disease to improve bradykinesia and rigidity rather than tremor. Orphenadrine is an antimuscarinic agent indicated in patients with Parkinson's disease where tremor predominates. Trifluoperazine is a piperazine antipsychotic that should be used with caution in patients with Parkinson's disease as its use may exacerbate the condition.

A77 C

Metronidazole is an antiprotozoal agent that, if taken concomitantly with alcohol, may result in a disulfiram-like reaction characterised by intense vasodilation, headache, tachycardia, sweating and vomiting.

A78 B

Salicylic acid is a keratolytic agent that removes layers of cornified skin cells. Treatment for corns, calluses and warts involves the application of salicylic acid at a concentration of 11–50%. Salicylic acid is contraindicated in allergic patients and its use should be avoided in diabetic patients.

Epidermabrasion refers to the physical process of removing the horny skin layer using a mechanical aid. It does not involve any pharmacological agents and is a safe and effective method for removing corns and calluses. Corns and calluses occurring in diabetic patients should be managed with care as diabetic patients may have a compromised peripheral circulation.

A79   E

Loperamide is an antidiarrhoeal drug indicated for use in adults and children over 12 years. Loperamide should not be administered in children under 4 years who have diarrhoea. Children are more sensitive to the occurrence of the side-effect of respiratory depression. Fluid and electrolyte replacement are first-line treatments in diarrhoea.

A80   B

Tardive dyskinesia is a chronic movement disorder characterised by uncontrolled facial movement disorders. Tardive dyskinesia is associated with the use of antipsychotics such as trifluoperazine.

A81   D

Beclometasone is a corticosteroid. Corticosteroids are used as prophylaxis in patients with asthma and therefore have no use in an acute attack. Bronchodilators acting as relievers are indicated for an acute attack. In asthma, patients are advised first to administer the bronchodilator, which acts very fast and then apply the corticosteroid, which has anti-inflammatory properties.

A82   E

Concomitant administration of diuretics and angiotensin-converting enzyme (ACE) inhibitors results in enhanced hypotensive effect. Blood pressure monitoring is required, therefore, if patients who are on diuretics are started on ACE inhibitors. The ACE inhibitor should be initiated in the evening to avoid falls due to hypotension.

A83   D

Codeine is a cough suppressant that can be used when an underlying cause for the cough cannot be identified and so the codeine is used to avoid the coughing from disturbing sleep. Being an antitussive it may lead to sputum retention. In the event of a known cause, e.g. a side-effect of a drug such as an ACE inhibitor, the use of the original drug should be reviewed rather than using a drug to counteract a side-effect.

A84   E

Clarithromycin is a derivative of erythromycin (macrolide). Advantages over erythromycin include lower frequency of gastrointestinal side-effects and lower dosage frequency. Clarithromycin is administered every 12 hours. As with all macrolides it should be used with caution in patients who are at risk of developing QT interval prolongation caused either by electrolyte imbalances or the concomitant use of other drugs.

A85   C

The use of imidazole antifungal agents such as econazole is the mainstay of treatment in vaginal thrush (candidiasis).

A86   B

When administered concomitantly, clarithromycin and the oral anticoagulant warfarin may interact, resulting in an enhanced anticoagulant effect and therefore increased risk of bleeding.

A87   B

Codeine may cause drowsiness and patients should be advised to avoid operating machinery and driving. Patients taking antibiotics should be advised to take the medicines at regular intervals and to complete the course of treatment prescribed.

A88 B

This combination product is an example of a combined hormone replacement therapy that increases the risk of stroke slightly and, with long-term use, increases the risk of ovarian cancer slightly. Hormone replacement therapy alleviates symptoms of menopause and can be used as a prophylaxis of osteoporosis.

A89 C

Patients on hormone replacement therapy such as the product prescribed are advised to take one tablet daily, starting subsequent courses without interval.

A90 B

Such a product is contraindicated in oestrogen-dependent carcinoma and thromboembolic disorders because of the oestrogen component. A history of migraine is not an absolute contraindication but requires administration with caution. Migraine is a side-effect associated with the oestrogen component.

A91 B

Combined hormone replacement therapy is also available as self-adhesive patches and creams.

A92 E

Amitriptyline is a tricylic antidepressant and these have antimuscarinic side-effects, such as urinary retention, blurred vision, dry mouth and sweating. They also tend to cause drowsiness.

A93 A

In this case the patient is advised to take two tablets three times daily.

A94 B

Tricylic antidepressants such as amitriptyline cause antimuscarinic side-effects, such as dry mouth and constipation. These antidepressants also tend to exhibit a time lag of about 3 weeks before the symptoms of depression are improved. Patients must be advised about the potential side-effects and that the drug may take some time to have an effect.

A95   A

Treatment for acne usually takes at least 3 months. In this case the patient must take one clindamycin capsule twice daily for 3 months.

A96   E

Clindamycin, which is active against Gram-positive aerobic organisms and Gram-negative anaerobes, may cause antibiotic-associated colitis.

A97   A

Glibenclamide is an oral antidiabetic agent (sulphonylurea). It acts by increasing insulin secretion and is therefore indicated in type 2 diabetes (non-insulin dependent) where there is pancreatic activity.

A98   B

Hypoglycaemic attacks may develop if the patient follows weight-reducing diets and skips meals. The patient is therefore advised to carry sweets, to be taken if signs of hypoglycaemia develop.

A99   C

Signs characteristic of hypoglycaemia include sweating, palpitations, pallor, tremor and weakness.

A100 C

Glibenclamide is a long-acting sulphonylurea and therefore may result in hypoglycaemic attacks, especially during the night. Gliclazide is a short-acting sulphonylurea, consequently presenting a lower risk of hypoglycaemic attacks.

Test 8

Questions

Questions 1–20

Directions: Each of the questions or incomplete statements is followed by five suggested answers. Select the best answer in each case.

Q1 AG is prescribed 1 L dextrose 5% over 6 hours to start at 8.00 am. After 5 hours — at which point, 650 mL have been infused — the amount is changed to 1 L normal saline over 12 hours. At midnight, 850 mL have been infused. AG's total intravenous fluid intake in the period 8.00 am to midnight is:

A ❑ 650 mL
B ❑ 850 mL
C ❑ 1000 mL
D ❑ 1500 mL
E ❑ 2000 mL

Q2 A woman with a body weight of 77 kg is prescribed dapsone 2 mg/kg daily. Dapsone is available as 50 mg tablets. The number of tablets to be dispensed for 30 days' supply is:

A ❑ 30
B ❑ 56
C ❑ 60
D ❑ 90
E ❑ 100

Q3   A patient is prescribed 3 L normal saline over 12 hours using a 5 drops/mL infusion set. The infusion rate in drops/minute is:

A   ❑ 5
B   ❑ 12
C   ❑ 15
D   ❑ 21
E   ❑ 25

Q4   The amount in grams of sodium bicarbonate that are contained in a 10 mL disposable syringe of 4.2% w/w sodium bicarbonate is:

A   ❑ 0.000 42
B   ❑ 0.004 2
C   ❑ 0.042
D   ❑ 0.42
E   ❑ 4.2

Q5   A stock solution is diluted to make a 1 in 5 strength solution. The amount in millilitres of the stock solution that is present in 250 mL of the resulting solution is:

A   ❑ 1
B   ❑ 25
C   ❑ 50
D   ❑ 250
E   ❑ 1250

Q6   Rhinocort Aqua delivers 64 µg of budesonide per dose and contains 120 doses. The amount of budesonide in mg per pack is:

A   ❑ 0.064
B   ❑ 7.68
C   ❑ 76.8
D   ❑ 768
E   ❑ 7680

Q7   Each sachet of Dioralyte contains 0.47 g sodium chloride and 0.30 g potassium chloride. The amount in millimoles of chloride in one sachet is (relative atomic mass of sodium = 23; chlorine = 35; potassium = 39):

A   ❑ 0.012
B   ❑ 0.12
C   ❑ 4.05
D   ❑ 8.10
E   ❑ 12.15

Q8   A patient has a serum potassium level of 6 mmol/L. The amount of potassium in milligrams in a 20 mL sample of the patient's serum is (relative atomic mass of potassium = 39):

A   ❑ 3.08
B   ❑ 4.68
C   ❑ 30.8
D   ❑ 46.80
E   ❑ 4680

Q9   The amount in millligrams of hydrocortisone required to prepare 30 g of hydrocortisone 0.1% w/w cream is:

A   ❑ 0.000 3
B   ❑ 0.003
C   ❑ 0.03
D   ❑ 0.3
E   ❑ 30

Q10   The amount in grams of a powder required to make 5 L of an aqueous solution at a concentration of 2% w/v of the anhydrous substance is (the powder contains 5% w/w moisture):

A ❑ 10
B ❑ 25
C ❑ 26.32
D ❑ 100
E ❑ 105

Q11   The volume in litres that can be produced of a 1:500 solution of chlorhexidine from 200 mL of a 4% solution of chlorhexidine is:

A ❑ 0.2
B ❑ 0.4
C ❑ 2
D ❑ 4
E ❑ 4000

Q12   Calculate the amount of drug in milligrams that is removed from the body in 24 hours. The drug has a clearance of 1.5 L/hour and the patient has a serum concentration of 2 mg/L:

A ❑ 0.072
B ❑ 3
C ❑ 36
D ❑ 48
E ❑ 72

Q13   The % concentration v/v of a 50 g cream that contains 1.25 g ketoprofen is:

A ❑ 0.02
B ❑ 0.2
C ❑ 1.25
D ❑ 2.5
E ❑ 25

Q14 A syringe pump is delivering voriconazole infusion 200 mg/50 mL at a rate of 2.5 mL/hour to a male patient with a body weight of 75 kg. The dose in µg/kg per hour that the patient is receiving is:

A   ❑ 0.13
B   ❑ 0.19
C   ❑ 10
D   ❑ 133
E   ❑ 188

Q15 The % v/v concentration of a solution of mivacurium 500 µg/mL is:

A   ❑ 0.000 5
B   ❑ 0.005
C   ❑ 0.05
D   ❑ 0.5
E   ❑ 50

Q16 Heparin is available as 5 mL vials containing 1000 units/mL. The number of heparin vials required to be able to give a loading dose of 75 units/kg to a female patient with a body weight of 85 kg is:

A   ❑ 0.5
B   ❑ 1
C   ❑ 2
D   ❑ 6
E   ❑ 7

Q17 A patient is receiving continuous insulin aspart 0.05 unit/mL in 0.9% sodium chloride at a rate of 5 mL/min. The amount of insulin units that the patient receives in 1 hour is:

A   ❑ 0.05
B   ❑ 5
C   ❑ 15
D   ❑ 30
E   ❑ 300

Q18   A patient is prescribed 40 mg furosemide in 500 mL Ringer's solution. Furosemide should be given at a rate not exceeding 4 mg/minute. The rate in millilitres per minute that should not be exceeded is:

A   ❑   0.08
B   ❑   0.32
C   ❑   0.5
D   ❑   10
E   ❑   50

Q19   The cost of 28 sachets of strontium ranelate 2 g is €47.12. Calculate the cost of treatment for 24 weeks:

A   ❑   47.12
B   ❑   141.36
C   ❑   282.72
D   ❑   599.10
E   ❑   848.16

Q20   A patient is prescribed flecainide 100 mg twice daily for 5 days and then 50 mg twice daily for 2 weeks. Flecainide is available as 50 mg tablets. The number of tablets to be dispensed is:

A   ❑   20
B   ❑   28
C   ❑   38
D   ❑   48
E   ❑   56

Questions 21–30

Directions: Each group of questions below consists of five lettered headings followed by a list of numbered questions. For each numbered question select the one heading that is most closely related to it. Each heading may be used once, more than once, or not at all.

Questions 21–23 concern the following drugs:

A   ❑ acetazolamide
B   ❑ mebeverine
C   ❑ ranitidine
D   ❑ tranexamic acid
E   ❑ zolmitriptan

Select, from A to E, which one of the above:

Q21   inhibits carbonic anhydrase

Q22   inhibits fibrinolysis

Q23   reduces intestinal motility

Questions 24–27 concern the following drugs:

A   ❑ guaiphenesin
B   ❑ ipratropium bromide
C   ❑ ranitidine
D   ❑ salbutamol
E   ❑ sodium cromoglicate

Select, from A to E, which one of the above:

Q24   blocks presynaptic muscarinic inhibition of acetylcholine release

Q25   is a direct-acting sympathomimetic

Q26   reduces parasympathetically induced mucus secretion

Q27   inhibits actions of histamine mediated by H_2 receptors

Questions 28–30 concern the following drugs:

A   ❏ acarbose
B   ❏ gliclazide
C   ❏ metformin
D   ❏ repaglinide
E   ❏ rosiglitazone

Select, from A to E, which one of the above is contraindicated in:

Q28   inflammatory bowel disease

Q29   history of heart failure

Q30   patients undergoing general anaesthesia

Questions 31–49

Directions: For each of the questions below, ONE or MORE of the responses is (are) correct. Decide which of the responses is (are) correct. Then choose:

A   ❑ if 1, 2 and 3 are correct
B   ❑ if 1 and 2 only are correct
C   ❑ if 2 and 3 only are correct
D   ❑ if 1 only is correct
E   ❑ if 3 only is correct

Directions summarised				
A	**B**	**C**	**D**	**E**
1, 2, 3	1, 2 only	2, 3 only	1 only	3 only

Q31   In polymorphism:

1   ❑ molecules arrange themselves in two or more different ways in the crystal
2   ❑ different X-ray diffraction patterns of polymorphs are produced
3   ❑ polymorphs exhibit the same physical and chemical properties

Q32   If the solubility of a drug substance is low:

1   ❑ the drug particles have a high surface-to-bulk ratio
2   ❑ micronisation may improve drug absorption
3   ❑ the dissolution rate *in vivo* may be the rate-controlling step in absorption

Q33   Drugs that are subject to oxidative degradation include:

1   ❏ phenothiazines
2   ❏ steroids
3   ❏ ascorbic acid

Q34   Polymers are used in pharmaceutical manufacturing as:

1   ❏ suspending agents
2   ❏ binding agents
3   ❏ emulsifying agents

Q35   In protein binding:

1   ❏ only albumin is involved
2   ❏ most drugs bind to a limited number of sites on the albumin molecule
3   ❏ binding is generally easily reversible

Questions 36–39 concern the following structure:

Q36   The structure represents a drug that:

1   ❑ includes an acetamide
2   ❑ contains two activating groups making the benzene ring highly reactive towards electrophilic aromatic substitution
3   ❑ is soluble in benzene

Q37   The drug:

1   ❑ is rapidly absorbed after oral administration
2   ❑ is primarily metabolised by the liver
3   ❑ may be oxidised

Q38   The drug is not contraindicated in:

1   ❑ asthmatic patients
2   ❑ patients with a history of hypertension
3   ❑ paediatric patients

Q39   In overdosage, symptoms that may occur include:

1   ❑ nausea
2   ❑ vomiting
3   ❑ right subcostal pain and tenderness

Questions 40–44 concern the following structure:

Q40 The structure represents a drug that presents a:

1 ❑ 3-keto group on ring A
2 ❑ 11 β-hydroxyl group on ring C
3 ❑ 17 α-hydroxyl group on ring D

Q41 Fluorination in this drug:

1 ❑ leads to an electron-withdrawing effect
2 ❑ increases lipophilicity
3 ❑ decreases activity

Q42 The drug should be used with caution in patients predisposed to:

1 ❑ hypertension
2 ❑ psychiatric reactions
3 ❑ osteoporosis

Q43 Indications for the use of the drug include:

1 ❑ ocular herpes simplex
2 ❑ congenital adrenal hyperplasia
3 ❑ eczema

Q44 Side-effects that may occur following systemic administration include:

1 ❑ dyspepsia
2 ❑ weight loss
3 ❑ decreased appetite

Questions 45–49 concern the following prescription:

Patient's name: . . . .

Diclofenac 50 mg tablets
1 tablet t.d.s.   m. 20 tablets
Cefuroxime 250 mg tablets
1 tablet b.d.   m. 10 tablets . . . .

Doctor's signature: . . . .

Q45   Diclofenac is:

1   ❏ a phenylacetic acid derivative
2   ❏ used as the sodium or potassium salt
3   ❏ may be used in breast-feeding mothers

Q46   Diclofenac may be administered:

1   ❏ orally as dispersible tablets
2   ❏ at a maximum oral daily dose not exceeding 150 mg
3   ❏ safely in a patient receiving venlafaxine

Q47   Cefuroxime is:

1   ❏ a third-generation cephalosporin
2   ❏ administered orally as the axetil salt
3   ❏ widely distributed in the body

Q48   Cefuroxime may be used in:

1   ❏ bacterial vaginosis
2   ❏ urinary tract infections
3   ❏ otitis media

Q49 In the event that diclofenac tablets are not available, product(s) that may be recommended to the prescriber include:

1 ❑ naproxen 500 mg b.d.
2 ❑ mefenamic acid 500 mg t.d.s.
3 ❑ co-codamol tablets t.d.s.

Questions 50–80

Directions: The following questions consist of a first statement followed by a second statement. Decide whether the first statement is true or false. Decide whether the second statement is true or false. Then choose:

A ❑ if both statements are true and the second statement is a *correct explanation* of the first statement
B ❑ if both statements are true but the second statement *is NOT a correct explanation* of the first statement
C ❑ if the first statement is true but the second statement is false
D ❑ if the first statement is false but the second statement is true
E ❑ if both statements are false

Directions summarised			
	First statement	**Second statement**	
A	True	True	Second statement is a *correct explanation* of the first
B	True	True	Second statement is *NOT a correct explanation* of the first
C	True	False	
D	False	True	
E	False	False	

Q50 Systemic use of chloramphenicol is reserved for life-threatening infections. Chloramphenicol may cause reversible aplastic anaemia.

Q51 Fluoroquinolones are generally not recommended for use in children. Fluoroquinolones may cause tendon inflammation and damage.

Q52 A patient who is taking metronidazole tablets should be advised to take tablets with or after food and to avoid alcoholic drink. When alcohol is consumed with metronidazole, the patient may present with acute psychoses or confusion.

Q53 Domperidone may be used to prevent motion sickness. Domperidone is a dopamine antagonist that acts at the chemoreceptor trigger zone.

Q54 Domperidone should not be used in patients receiving co-careldopa. Domperidone is commonly associated with the occurrence of extrapyramidal effects.

Q55 Loperamide is a synthetic opioid analogue that increases gut motility. Loperamide should be avoided in patients with active ulcerative colitis.

Q56 Acetone is a clear, colourless volatile liquid with a characteristic odour. Inhalation of acetone may cause central nervous system depression.

Q57 Pilocarpine is a tertiary amine parasympathomimetic agent that is mainly used in the treatment of glaucoma. Pilocarpine is commonly administered with timolol eye drops.

Q58 Patients receiving pilocarpine eye drops should be advised that driving at night may be affected. Administration of pilocarpine may cause blurred vision, headache and brow ache as side-effects.

Q59 Hepatitis B vaccination is recommended to individuals with haemophilia. Hepatitis B vaccination requires one single dose.

Q60   When a patient who is receiving atenolol is started on terazosin, there is an increased risk of first-dose hypotension. Terazosin is an alpha-adrenoceptor agonist which causes vasodilatation.

Q61   Carbamazepine has anti-epileptic and psychotropic properties. Carbamazepine is related chemically to the tricyclic antidepressants.

Q62   Patients receiving carbamazepine should be advised how to recognise signs of blood disorders. Carbamazepine should be withdrawn if leucopenia that is severe, progressive or associated with clinical symptoms occurs.

Q63   When dispensing carbamazepine tablets it is prudent to avoid changing the formulation. Carbamazepine is absorbed slowly and erratically after oral administration.

Q64   Initiating carbamazepine therapy in a patient receiving oral contraceptives decreases the contraceptive effect. Carbamazepine decreases the metabolism of oestrogens and progestogens.

Q65   All benzodiazepines have similar pharmacological profiles. Benzodiazepines have similar pharmacodynamic spectra and pharmacokinetic properties.

Q66   Hypnotic doses of diazepam may cause hyperventilation in patients with severe chronic obstructive pulmonary disease. Diazepam causes central nervous system depression.

Q67   Diazepam may be used in status epilepticus. Diazepam has a long half-life and exhibits rapid entry into the brain.

Q68   Benzodiazepines with a short elimination half-life present a less severe withdrawal after drug discontinuation than drugs with a long elimination half-life. Symptoms of benzodiazepine withdrawal syndrome include anxiety, depression, insomnia and headache.

Q69 At therapeutic doses the occurrence of a negative inotropic effect with amlodipine is rarely seen. Amlodipine has greater selectivity for vascular smooth muscle than for myocardium.

Q70 Amlodipine should not be prescribed in patients who are receiving valsartan. Both amlodipine and valsartan may cause dizziness.

Q71 Patients receiving alendronic acid tablets should be advised to swallow tablet whole with plenty of water. Absorption of alendronic acid is increased leading to higher frequency of side-effects if tablet is swallowed with drinks containing milk.

Q72 Glucosamine is a natural substance that is present in tendons and ligaments. Glucosamine is used for the symptomatic relief of mild-to-moderate osteoarthritis in combination with chondroitin.

Q73 Glucosamine should be used with care in patients with impaired glucose tolerance. Glucosamine may cause nausea, abdominal pain and indigestion as side-effects.

Q74 Patients using oral rehydration salts should be advised that after reconstitution, any unused solution should be discarded no later than 1 hour after preparation unless stored in a refrigerator. Oral rehydration solutions should be slightly hypo-osmolar.

Q75 Use of ibandronic acid leads to an increase in the bone mineral density at the spine. Ibandronic acid interferes with bone mineralization and results in an overall increase in bone remodelling and bone turnover.

Q76 Levothyroxine sodium is the synthetically prepared sodium salt of the natural isomer of thyroid hormone. Levothyroxine sodium tablets are unstable and require administration on an empty stomach.

Q77   When starting levothyroxine, a baseline ECG is recommended. The baseline ECG is used to distinguish underlying myocardial ischaemia from changes induced by hypothyroidism.

Q78   Levothyroxine is contraindicated in patients with a history of myocardial infarction. Levothyroxine may cause palpitations and tachycardia as side-effects.

Q79   Tamoxifen is an oestrogen-receptor antagonist that is only effective as adjuvant endocrine therapy of early breast cancer in postmenopausal women. Tamoxifen is given by mouth and treatment should not exceed 1 year.

Q80   Women receiving tamoxifen should be advised to have routine gynaecological monitoring. Uterine fibroids and endometrial changes may occur with tamoxifen.

Questions 81–100

Directions: Read the statement or patient request and follow the instructions.

Questions 81–83:

Extrapyramidal symptoms may occur as a side-effect of antipsychotic drugs.

Put the following in order of precipitation of extrapyramidal symptoms, assigning 1 to the drug most likely to induce them and 3 to the drug least likely to induce this side-effect.

Q81   chlorpromazine

Q82   olanzapine

Q83   prochlorperazine

Questions 84–86:

Put the following adverse effects of fluticasone aqueous nasal spray in order of occurrence, assigning 1 to the side-effect that occurs most commonly and 3 to the side-effect that occurs least commonly.

Q84   bronchospasms

Q85   irritation of nose

Q86   raised intraocular pressure

Questions 87–89:

A client asks for a salicylic acid gel he is buying for his mother for the removal of corns and calluses.

Put the following counselling points by the pharmacist in order of relevance, assigning 1 to the information that is most important to be presented to the patient and 3 to the information that is least relevant to the patient.

Q87   to protect surrounding skin with petroleum jelly

Q88   not to use if the patient is diabetic

Q89   to rub the surface gently with a file or pumice stone daily

Questions 90–95:

A patient presents with symptoms of blepharitis.

For the following drugs, place your order of preference, assigning 1 to the product that should be recommended as first choice and 6 to the product that should be recommended as a last choice.

Q90   chloramphenicol eye drops

Q91   ciprofloxacin tablets

Q92   dexamethasone eye drops

Q93   fusidic acid eye drops

Q94   gentamicin eye ointment

Q95   gentamicin and betamethasone eye drops

Questions 96–100:

Put the following diagnostic tests in order of relevance for the management of a diabetic patient on insulin therapy, assigning 1 to the test that should be recommended as first choice and 5 to the test that should be recommended as a last choice.

Q96   blood glucose measurement

Q97   blood cholesterol and triglycerides measurement

Q98   glycosylated haemoglobin

Q99   urinalysis for glucose

Q100   urinalysis for leukocytes and nitrites

Test 8

Answers

A1   D

The patient was infused 650 mL of dextrose 5% and 850 mL of normal saline giving a total of 1500 mL between 8.00 am and midnight.

A2   D

The patient's daily dose is 154 mg (2 mg × 77 kg). Dapsone tablets are available as 50 mg so the patient requires 3 tablets of dapsone 50 mg on a daily basis. Hence 90 tablets (3 × 30 days) of dapsone 50 mg should be dispensed to the patient.

A3   D

The patient should be given 3000 mL over 720 minutes (12 hours × 60 minutes). Since 5 drops make 1 mL then 15 000 drops (3000 mL × 5 drops) are required for 3000 mL. Hence 15 000 drops should be infused over 720 minutes at a rate of 20.8 (15 000/720) or 21 drops/minute.

A4   D

There are 4.2 g of sodium bicarbonate in 100 mL; in 10 mL of solution there are 0.42 g (4.2 × 10/100).

A5   C

A 1 : 5 strength solution is 50 (250/5) mL : 250 mL resulting solution.

A6   B

One pack of Rhinocort Acqua delivers a total dose of 7680 µg (64 µg × 120 doses), equivalent to 7.68 mg (7680/1000).

A7   E

The molar mass of sodium chloride (NaCl) is 58 (23 + 35). The molar mass of potassium chloride (KCl) is 74 (39 + 35). The number of moles is weight (g)/molar mass. For NaCl: 0.47g/58 = 0.008 moles and for KCl: 0.30g/74 = 0.004 moles. Total moles of chloride are 0.012 moles (0.008 + 0.004), which is equivalent to 12 millimoles (0.012 × 1000).

A8   B

A concentration of 6 mmol/L is equivalent to 0.006 moles/L. The amount of potassium/L is 0.234 g (0.006 × 39); 0.234 g is equivalent to 234 mg/1000 mL. In 20 mL, the amount of potassium is 4.68 mg (234/1000 × 20).

A9   E

A concentration of 0.1% w/w means 0.1 g in 100 g. In order to prepare 30 g of 0.1% w/w, 0.03 g are required (0.1 × 30/100); 0.03 g is equivalent to 30 mg.

A10   E

A 2% w/v solution is equivalent to 2 g in 100 mL. Hence in 5 litres, 100 g of powder are required (5000 mL × 2 g/100 mL). However, a 100 g of powder would also contain 5 g (5 g in 100 g = 5% w/w) of moisture, so to counteract, you need 105 g of powder.

A11   D

A 4% solution means 4 mL of chlorhexidine in 100 mL. Hence a 200 mL solution means 8 mL (0.008 litres) of the solute. To prepare a 1 : 500 solution, 0.008 litres : 4 litres (0.008 × 500).

A12   E

In 24 hours a total of 36 L are removed (1.5 L × 24 hours). Given that the serum concentration is 2 mg/L, a total of 72 mg (36 L × 2) are removed.

A13   D

An amount of 50 g cream contains 1.25 g ketoprofen, therefore 100 g cream contains 2.5 g (100 × 1.25/50) which is equivalent to 2.5% v/v.

A14   D

In 50 mL there are 200 mg voriconazole, in 2.5 mL there are 10 mg (200 × 2.5/50). In 1 hour 10 mg are delivered, which is equivalent to 0.133 mg/kg per hour (10 mg/75 kg), that is, 133 μg/kg per hour.

A15   C

An amount of 50 000 μg (500 μg × 100 mL) are in 100 mL equivalent to 0.05 g in 100 mL. The % v/v is 0.05%.

A16   C

The total dose required is 6375 units (75 units × 85 kg); 1000 units are contained in 1 mL and 6375 units are contained in 6.375 mL (6375/1000). Given that each vial contains 5 mL, two vials are required to give the total loading dose.

A17   C

The patient receives 15 units in 1 hour (0.05 units × 5 mL × 60 minutes).

A18   E

In 500 mL of Ringer's solution, 40 mg furosemide are found, 4 mg furosemide are found in 50 mL (4 × 500/40) of solution. Hence the infusion rate should be 50 mL/minute.

A19   C

Strontium ranelate is administered as 2 g once daily. In 24 weeks, the patient would require 6 packs of 28 sachets. If one pack of 28 sachets costs €47.12, 6 packs cost €282.72 (47.12 × 6).

A20 D

For the 100 mg, twice daily, 5-day regimen, the patient requires 20 tablets (2 × 2 × 5). For the 50 mg, twice-daily 14-day regimen, the patient requires 28 tablets (2 × 14). The total number of tablets to be dispensed is 48 (20 + 28) tablets.

A21 A

Acetazolamide is a carbonic anhydrase inhibitor that is administered orally for the treatment of glaucoma. Topical carbonic anhydrase inhibitors include dorzolamide and brinzolamide. Carbonic anhydrase inhibitors reduce the production of aqueous humour, thereby reducing intraocular pressure. They can be used alone or in addition to beta-blocker therapy in glaucoma patients.

A22 D

Tranexamic acid inhibits fibrinolysis. It is used to prevent bleeding or to treat bleeding problems in various conditions and in the management of menorrhagia.

A23 B

Mebeverine is an antispasmodic that reduces gastric and intestinal motility by direct relaxation of the intestinal smooth muscle. It can be used to relieve pain in irritable bowel syndrome and diverticular disease. Like all antispasmodics, mebeverine is contraindicated in paralytic ileus.

A24 B

Ipratropium is classified as an anticholinergic because it blocks acetylcholine release. It is indicated in asthma and chronic obstructive pulmonary disease and is available for inhalation.

A25 D

Salbutamol is a beta-adrenoreceptor agonist that is used in asthma or chronic obstructive pulmonary disease in order to exert bronchodilation. Side-effects of beta-adrenoreceptor agonists include tremor, tachycardia, headache and nervous tension.

A26   B

Being an anticholinergic, ipratropium interrupts the parasympathetic activities including the blocking of muscarinic receptors in the lung, resulting in an inhibition of bronchoconstriction and of mucus secretion.

A27   C

Ranitidine is a histamine receptor antagonist. It acts essentially on the H_2 receptor and blocks acid production. Ranitidine is used in the treatment and prevention of ulcers, NSAID-induced ulcers, Zollinger–Ellison syndrome and gastro-oesophageal reflux disease.

A28   A

Acarbose is an intestinal α-glucosidase inhibitor that delays digestion and absorption of starch and sucrose. It is used in diabetes mellitus and is contraindicated in inflammatory bowel disease.

A29   E

Rosiglitazone, a thiazolinedione used to treat diabetes mellitus, is contraindicated in patients with heart failure especially if taken in combination with insulin.

A30   C

Metformin is a biguanide used to treat diabetes mellitus. It is contraindicated in patients undergoing general anaesthesia since anaesthesia can interfere with renal function. The risk of lactic acidosis associated with metformin increases in patients with renal impairment. Metformin should be stopped before and during surgery where anaesthesia is indicated. Metformin should only be restarted after the renal function has returned to normal.

A31   B

When polymorphism occurs, the molecules arrange themselves in two or more different ways in the crystal: either they may be packed differently in the crystal lattice, or there may be differences in the orientation or the conformation of the molecules at the lattice site. These variations cause differences in X-ray diffraction patterns of the polymorphs and this technique is one of the main methods in detecting them. The polymorphs have different physical and chemical properties.

A32   C

For poorly soluble drugs, the digestive absorption depends on their rate of dissolution. Decreasing the particle size of these drugs to increase the surface-to-bulk ratio improves their rate of dissolution. Fine-grinding mills are used to micronise powders.

A33   B

Steroids and sterols represent an important class of drugs that are susceptible to oxidative degradation through the possession of alkene moieties. The oxidation of phenothiazines forms the sulfoxide moiety.

A34   A

Polymers have a number of applications in the development of formulations. They have the properties of suspending agents, binding agents and emulsifying agents. They are included in formulations for the production of tablets, suspensions and emulsions. Polymers can be used as film coatings to disguise the unpleasant taste of a drug, to enhance drug stability and to modify drug release characteristics in modified-release preparations.

A35   C

Drug–protein binding is the reversible interaction of drugs with different proteins in plasma. Albumin is not the exclusive protein involved. Drugs bind to specific sites on the protein.

A36   B

The figure represents the chemical structure for paracetamol, which includes the N-(4-hydroxyphenyl) acetamide, derived from the interaction of *p*-aminophenol and an aqueous solution of acetic anhydride. The structure has two activating groups that make the benzene ring highly reactive toward electrophilic aromatic substitution.

A37   A

After oral administration, paracetamol is completely absorbed from the gastrointestinal tract with peak plasma concentrations being reached in less than an hour. The drug is eliminated by conjugation with glucoronic acid in the liver. The chemical structure is liable to oxidation.

A38   A

Paracetamol can be used in asthmatic patients (as opposed to non-steroidal anti-inflammatory drugs), in patients with a history of hypertension and in paediatric patients.

A39   A

The intermediate metabolites formed during the biotransformation in the liver are believed to be responsible for the hepatoxicity that results in overdosage. Nausea and vomiting are early features of poisoning. With time, hepatic necrosis develops and is often associated with the onset of right subcostal pain and tenderness.

A40   A

Betamethasone is the steroid represented by this structure. It is composed of a 3-keto group on ring A, an 11β-hydroxyl group and a 17α-hydroxyl group on ring C and D respectively.

A41   D

Betamethasone is a fluorinated steroid. Fluorination is substitution with an electron-attracting group and increases potency.

A42   A

Steroids have mineralocorticoid and glucocorticoid effects. Betamethasone has little, if any, mineralocorticoid effect. However, it should be used with caution in patients predisposed to hypertension since mineralocorticoid effects may lead to sodium and water retention and an increase in blood pressure. When used systemically, especially at high doses, steroid therapy is associated with a risk of psychiatric reactions such as euphoria, irritability, mood lability and sleep disorders. Glucocorticoid side-effects include diabetes and osteoporosis.

A43   C

Betamethasone, as with all steroids, is used to suppress inflammatory reactions. It can be used topically or systemically. Indications for its use include eczema, asthma and congenital adrenal hyperplasia. It is contraindicated in ocular herpes simplex and in the 'red eye syndrome' since it may clear the symptoms while not addressing the infective component of the underlying condition.

A44   D

Following systemic administration, side-effects to be expected are related to the mineralocorticoid and glucocorticoid effects, and include gastrointestinal effects (dyspepsia), neuropsychiatric effects and ophthalmic effects. Increased appetite and weight gain may occur as a result of corticosteroid therapy. In fact systemic use of corticosteroids is considered in palliative care because it increases patient's appetite and feeling of well-being. Risk of occurrence of side-effects is related to dosage use and duration of treatment.

A45   A

Diclofenac is a phenylacetic acid derivative, non-steroidal anti-inflammatory drug. It is available as the potassium and sodium salts. Potassium salts are slightly more soluble than the sodium salts. Diclofenac can be used in breast-feeding mothers since the amount that passes through breast milk is too small to be harmful to the baby. However, diclofenac is contraindicated in pregnancy, especially during the last trimester.

A46   B

Diclofenac is available as dispersible tablets, tablets, gel, suppositories and for intravenous or intramuscular injection. The maximum dose of diclofenac administered via any route is 150 mg. As with other non-steroidal anti-inflammatory drugs, concomitant use in patients receiving venlafaxine increases the risk of bleeding.

A47   C

Cefuroxime is a second-generation cephalosporin. Orally, cefuroxime is available as the prodrug, cefuroxime axetil. Cefuroxime is very well absorbed from the gastrointestinal tract and widely distributed in the body.

A48   C

Cefuroxime is indicated to treat infections of bacterial origin such as urinary tract infections, otitis media and upper respiratory tract infections. Bacterial vaginosis is likely to be treated with metronidazole and clindamycin.

A49   B

Alternative products to diclofenac include naproxen and mefenamic acid, both of which are non-steroidal anti-inflammatory drugs. Co-codamol is a mixture of the opioid analgesic codeine and paracetamol and it does not possess the anti-inflammatory component. It may be used in pain management either where NSAIDs are contraindicated or in patients who are intolerant to the effects of NSAIDs.

A50   A

The systemic use of chloramphenicol is reserved only for life-threatening infections where other anti-microbial therapy has failed or is inadequate, since chloramphenicol may cause reversible aplastic anaemia as a side-effect.

A51   A

Fluoroquinolones are contraindicated in children because they can cause irreversible tendon inflammation and damage. They should be used with caution in the elderly population. The risk is increased if fluoroquinolones are administered with corticosteroids.

A52   A

Metronidazole and alcohol interact resulting in a disulfiram-type reaction, which may present with acute psychoses and confusion leading to lethal consequences. Patients are therefore strongly advised not to consume alcohol during treatment with metronidazole and to take tablets with or after food.

A53   D

Domperidone is a dopamine antagonist that acts on the chemoreceptor trigger zone. It can therefore be used as an anti-emetic in nausea and vomiting, for example, to counteract side-effects of cytotoxic therapy and to treat nausea associated with dopaminergic drugs used in Parkinson's disease. Unlike hyoscine butlybromide and antihistamines, domperidone is ineffective in motion sickness.

A54   E

Domperidone is used in combination with antiparkinsonian drugs to counteract the nausea and vomiting caused by the latter. Since it does not readily cross the blood–brain barrier, it is not associated with extra-pyramidal effects and is less likely to cause dystonia than metoclopromide and phenothiazines.

A55   D

Loperamide is an opioid analogue that binds to the opiate gut receptors, thereby decreasing intestinal motility and increasing transit time. Loperamide is contraindicated in patients with active ulcerative colitis and children under 4 years. It is used in the treatment of diarrhoea.

A56   B

Acetone is a clear, colourless volatile liquid, which is also flammable. Acetone is a ketone and has a characteristic odour. It is miscible with water and alcohol. Its inhalation can lead to depression of the central nervous system.

A57   B

Pilocarpine is classified as a tertiary amine that has parasympathomimetic activity. When administered as eye drops, it causes pupillary constriction or miosis and is therefore indicated in the treatment of glaucoma. In glaucoma, multiple-drug therapy may be necessary to achieve the desired intraocular control. Pilocarpine may be used in combination with topical beta-blockers such as timolol.

A58   A

All patients receiving pilocarpine eye drops should be advised to be careful if driving at night since pilocarpine may cause blurred vision. Other side-effects include headache and brow ache secondary to ciliary spasms.

A59   C

Hepatitis B vaccine schedule consists of three injections given at time 0, 1 month after the first injection and a third injection given 6 months after the first injection. Patients at high risk are given a booster after 5 years to maintain the immunity profile. Patients receiving blood transfusions, haemophilia patients, patients with chronic liver disease, and haemodialysis patients are among the high-risk patients who should be vaccinated.

A60   C

Terazosin is an alpha-adrenoreceptor blocker that causes vasodilation and is used in the management of hypertension and benign prostatic hypertrophy. Beta-blockers and alpha-blockers can interact to induce hypotension since both act to reduce the blood pressure. Patients already on beta-blockers and who are started on alpha-blockers such as terazosin should be advised to take the terazosin dose at night to reduce the implications (falls) of first-dose hypotension.

A61   B

Carbamazepine is an anti-epileptic with psychotropic properties. It is chemically related to tricyclic antidepressants. Its uses include the treatment of epilepsy, trigeminal neuralgia, phantom limb and manic-depressive psychosis resistant to lithium therapy.

A62   A

Side-effects of carbamazepine include blood disorders such as thrombo-cytopenia, leucopenia, aplastic anaemia and agranulocytosis. Patients are therefore advised to stop treatment and contact a healthcare provider if they develop symptoms of sore throat, fever, rash, mouth ulcers, bleeding or bruising.

A63   A

Carbamazepine is slowly absorbed and tends to exhibit erratic absorption following oral administration. Hence, when dispensing repeat prescriptions for carbamazepine, it is advisable to avoid changing the formulation of carbamazepine.

A64   C

Carbamazepine interacts with oral contraceptives. Carbamazepine increases the metabolism of oestrogens and progestogens resulting in a decrease in the plasma concentration of oestrogens and progestogens. This in turn brings about a decrease in the contraceptive level provided.

A65   C

Benzodiazepines have similar pharmacological properties and are used in anxiety and insomnia. The choice of which benzodiazepine to use usually lies with the pharmacodynamic and pharmacokinetic properties, which vary across the class. For example, diazepam, flurazepam and nitrazepam have a prolonged duration of action whereas lorazepam and temazepam have a shorter duration of action.

A66   D

Diazepam can cause central nervous system depression. It may cause respiratory depression in overdosage but, at hypnotic doses, the risk of hyperventilation in patients with severe chronic obstructive pulmonary disease is minimal.

A67   B

Diazepam may be used in status epilepticus where it is administered intravenously. However, there is a risk of thrombophlebitis. Diazepam has a long half-life and it is rapidly absorbed into the brain.

A68   D

Benzodiazepines with a short half-life are excreted more rapidly than benzodiazepines with a long half-life and hence the risk of severe withdrawal side-effects is higher. Withdrawal symptoms include anxiety, depression, insomnia, headache and hallucinations.

A69   A

Amlodipine is a calcium-channel blocker that blocks the intracellular movement of calcium ions and hence slows the contractility of the myocardium and relaxes the vascular smooth muscle. The negative inotropic effects are rarely seen at therapeutic doses since amlodipine has a greater selectivity for vascular smooth muscle than for the myocardium.

A70   D

Calcium-channel blockers such as amlodipine can be used in patients receiving angiotensin-receptor blockers such as valsartan for the treatment of hypertension and angina. Side-effects common to both drugs include dizziness and hypotension.

A71   C

Oral administration of alendronic acid may cause gastrointestinal irritation. Patients are advised to swallow the tablets whole with plenty of water while standing or at least while in a sitting position. Concomitant administration of alendronic acid and calcium-containing products such as milk leads to decreased absorption of the alendronic acid and hence ineffectiveness.

A72   B

Glucosamine is an amino sugar derivative occurring naturally in healthy tendons, ligaments and cartilage. Its use has been shown to be effective in the symptomatic relief of osteoarthritis, especially in combination with chondroitin, also a derivative of cartilage.

A73   B

Being an amino sugar derivative, glucosamine should be used cautiously in patients with impaired glucose tolerance. Side-effects of glucosamine include nausea, abdominal pain and indigestion.

A74   B

Oral rehydration salts should be reconstituted with water. Patients are advised to put the reconstituted solution in the fridge or else it should be used up to 1 hour after reconstitution. Oral rehydration solution should be slightly hypo-osmolar to decrease the electrolyte and water loss from the intestines.

A75   C

Ibandronic acid is classified as a bisphosphonate and is used in the management of osteoporosis. It acts selectively on the bone mass, decreasing the osteoclast activity and hence resulting in an increase in bone mass, including the spine cavity.

A76   C

Levothyroxine is the synthetic sodium salt of the natural isomer of thyroid hormone. Levothyroxine is administered orally and is usually taken with breakfast to mimic the body's release and to avoid possible insomnia.

A77   A

Levothyroxine can induce arrythmias and hence a baseline electrocardiogram is recommended for eventual comparison. A baseline ECG can also be used to distinguish underlying myocardial ischaemia from changes induced by hypothyroidism in a newly diagnosed patient.

A78   D

Levothryoxine is contraindicated in thryotoxicosis but not in patients with a past history of myocardial infarction. Levothyroxine can cause palpitations, tachycardia, arrhythmias, restlessness, excitability and insomnia as side-effects. It should be used with caution in patients with cardiovascular disorders, including those with a past history of myocardial infarction; a lower dose should be used as a starting dose.

A79   E

Tamoxifen is an oestrogen-receptor antagonist effective in premenopausal, perimenopausal and postmenopausal women with early breast cancer. Aromatase inhibitors, such as anastrazole, may be used only in post-menopausal women. Tamoxifen is administered as tablets. Treatment with tamoxifen is usually given for at least 5 years.

A80   A

The administration of tamoxifen necessitates routine gynaecological monitoring since uterine fibroids and endometrial changes may occur with its use. Prior to starting treatment, patients should be informed of the small risk of endometrial cancer associated with tamoxifen therapy.

A81–83

Prochlorperazine is a potent phenothiazine antipsychotic drug that is associated with a high risk of extrapyramidal side-effects, a low degree of sedation and of antimuscarinic side-effects. Chlorpromazine is less likely to induce extrapyramidal side-effects but has increased risks of inducing sedation and antimuscarinic side-effects. Olanzapine is classified as an atypical antipsychotic having characteristically much fewer incidences of extrapyramidal side-effects. It is however associated with increased risk of stroke in elderly patients.

A81   2

A82   3

A83   1

A84–86

The most common side-effects to nasal administration of fluticasone are local reactions, including irritation of the nose and throat and epistaxis. Steroids may cause a raised intraocular pressure or glaucoma. Hypersensitivity reactions, including occurrence of bronchospasms, have been reported.

A84   3

A85   1

A86   2

A87–89

It is important to check that a patient presenting with a foot problem does not have diabetes. Diabetic patients are at an increased risk of developing infections because of injury from the keratolytic action of salicylic acid. Patient should be advised to apply petroleum jelly to the skin surrounding the area where salicylic acid will be applied. Petroleum jelly protects the skin from the irritation caused by the salicylic acid. Using a file or pumice stone to gently rub away the surface of the corn or calluses helps to remove them.

A87   2

A88   1

A89   3

A90–95

Blepharitis is a topical inflammation of the eyelid margins that should be treated using topical antibacterial agents. Gentamicin eye ointment is preferred to the fusidic acid drops since the ointment is a better formulation to be used where the condition involves the eyelid margins. Chloramphenicol eye drops is the third option since it is an antibiotic with a wider spectrum of activity. A combination of corticosteroid and antibiotic is not recommended because of the side-effects associated with the steroid. The use of oral tablets is not usually recommended since blepharitis can easily be managed with topical drops. The use of dexamethasone eye drops, monotherapy steroid, could clear the inflammation but mask persistence of infection.

A90   3

A91   5

A92   6

A93   2

A94   1

A95   4

A96–100

Diabetic patients should be educated and advised to check regularly their blood glucose level. These patients have an increased risk of cardiovascular-related morbidity and mortality and therefore blood cholesterol and triglyceride levels should be monitored. The glycosylated haemoglobin also known as HbA1C gives an indication of the blood glucose levels over the previous 3 months. Urinalysis for glucose is not an accurate test for checking blood glucose levels since there are a lot of variables that may interfere with the test. Urinalysis for leukocytes and nitrites will indicate the presence or absence of a bacterial infection and is not recommended as a regular test for diabetic patients unless a urinary tract infection is suspected.

A96   1

A97   2

A98   3

A99   4

A100   5

Bibliography

Azzopardi LM (2000). *Validation Instruments for Community Pharmacy: Pharmaceutical Care for the Third Millennium.* Binghamton, New York: Pharmaceutical Products Press.

Brunton LL, Lazo SJ, Parker KL eds (2006). *Goodman & Gilman's The Pharmacological Basis of Therapeutics*, 11th edn. New York: McGraw-Hill.

Edwards C, Stillman P (2006). *Minor Illness or Major Disease? The clinical pharmacist in the community*, 4th edn. London: Pharmaceutical Press.

Greene RJ, Harris ND (2008). *Pathology and Therapeutics for Pharmacists: a Basis for Clinical Pharmacy Practice*, 3rd edn. London: Pharmaceutical Press.

Harman RJ, ed (2000). *Handbook of Pharmacy Health-Education*, 2nd edn. London: Pharmaceutical Press.

Harman RJ, Mason P, eds (2002). *Handbook of Pharmacy Healthcare: Diseases and Patient Advice*, 2nd edn. London: Pharmaceutical Press.

Joint Formulary Committee, ed (2009). *British National Formulary*. London: Pharmaceutical Press.

Mosby's Dictionary of Medicine, Nursing & Health Professions, 8th edn (2009). St Louis, Missouri: Mosby.

Nathan A (2006). *Non-prescription Medicines*, 3rd edn. London: Pharmaceutical Press.

Pagana KD, Pagana TJ (1998). *Mosby's Manual of Diagnostic and Laboratory Tests*. St Louis, Missouri: Mosby.

Snell M, ed (2008). *Medicines, Ethics and Practice: a guide for pharmacists and pharmacy technicians*, 32nd rev edn. London: Royal Pharmaceutical Society of Great Britain.

Sweetman SC, ed (2006). *Martindale: the Complete Drug Reference*, 35th edn. London: Pharmaceutical Press.

Taylor LM (2002). *Pharmacy Preregistration Handbook: a survival guide*, 2nd edn. London: Pharmaceutical Press.

Appendix A

Proprietary (trade) names and equivalent generic names

The proprietary names used in this book can be found in Martindale: the Complete Drug Reference, *although not all are listed in the* British National Formulary.

Actifed	triprolidine, pseudoephedrine
Actifed Compound Linctus	triprolidine, pseudoephedrine, dextromethorphan
Actonel	risedronate
Adalat	nifedipine
Aldactone	spironolactone
Alka-Seltzer	aspirin, citric acid, sodium bicarbonate
Alupent	orciprenaline
Amoxil	amoxicillin
Anadin Extra	aspirin, paracetamol, caffeine
Arthrotec	diclofenac, misoprostol
Aspro	aspirin
Ativan	lorazepam
Atarax	hydroxyzine
Augmentin	co-amoxiclav (amoxicillin, clavulanic acid)
Avandia	rosiglitazone
Avomine	promethazine
Bactroban	mupirocin
Beechams Hot Lemon and Honey	paracetamol, ascorbic acid, phenylephrine
Betadine	povidone-iodine
Betnovate	betamethasone
Bezalip	bezafibrate
Bonviva	ibandronic acid
Buccastem	prochlorperazine
Buscopan	hyoscine butylbromide

Buspar	buspirone
Byetta	exenatide
Canesten	clotrimazole
Canesten HC	clotrimazole, hydrocortisone
Cardura	doxazosin
Cerumol	arachis oil, paradichlorobenzene, chlorobutanol
Cilest	ethinylestradiol, norgestimate
Ciproxin	ciprofloxacin
Circadin	melatonin
Cirrus	cetirizine, pseudoephedrine
Citramag	magnesium carbonate, citric acid
Clarinase	loratadine, pseudoephedrine
Clarityn	loratadine
Colofac	mebeverine
Corsodyl	chlorhexidine
Coversyl	perindopril
Cozaar	losartan
Cytotec	misoprostol
Daktacort	miconazole, hydrocortisone
Daktarin	miconazole
Dalacin	clindamycin
Day Nurse	paracetamol, phenylpropanolamine, dextromethorphan
Deltacortril	prednisolone
Dermovate	clobetasol
Diamox	acetazolamide
Didronel PMO	disodium etidronate, calcium carbonate
Difflam	benzydamine
Diflucan	fluconazole
Dioralyte	sodium chloride, sodium bicarbonate, potassium chloride, citric acid, glucose
Dovonex	calcipotriol

Drapolene	benzalkonium chloride, cetrimide
Dulco-lax	bisacodyl
Duphalac	lactulose
E45	light liquid paraffin, white soft paraffin, hypoallergenic hydrous wool fat (lanolin)
Elidel	pimecrolimus
Emadine	emedastine
Engerix B	hepatitis B surface antigen
Erythroped	erythromycin
Euglucon	glibenclamide
Eurax	crotamiton
Exelon	rivastigmine
Ezetrol	ezetimibe
Feldene	piroxicam
Flagyl	metronidazole
Flixotide	fluticasone
Flixonase	fluticasone
Fluarix	influenza vaccine
Fucicort	fusidic acid, betamethasone
Fucidin	fusidic acid
Fucidin H	fusidic acid, hydrocortisone
Fybogel	ispaghula husk
Gardasil	human papilloma virus vaccine (quadrivalent vaccine)
Gaviscon	oral suspension: calcium carbonate, alginate, sodium bicarbonate; tablets: alginic acid, aluminium hydroxide, magnesium trisilicate, sodium bicarbonate
Guttalax	sodium picosulfate
Gyno-Daktarin	miconazole
Havrix	formaldehyde-inactivated hepatitis A virus
Heminevrin	clomethiazole

Ikorel	nicorandil
Imodium	loperamide
Inderal	propranolol
Indocid	indometacin
Isordil	isosorbide dinitrate
Istin	amlodipine
Karvol	levomenthol, chlorobutanol, pine oils, terpineol, thymol
Kay-Cee-L	potassium chloride
Ketek	telithromycin
Klaricid	clarithromycin
Kwells	hyoscine hydrobromide
Lamisil	terbinafine
Lanoxin	digoxin
Lantus	insulin glargine
Largactil	chlorpromazine
Lasilix	furosemide
Lescol	fluvastatin
Lipobase	fatty cream base
Livial	tibolone
Losec	omeprazole
Lucentis	ranibizumab
Maalox	aluminium hydroxide, magnesium hydroxide
Macrodantin	nitrofurantoin
Migril	ergotamine, cyclizine, caffeine
Mobic	meloxicam
Molcer	docusate sodium
Motilium	domperidone
Naprosyn	naproxen
Nasonex	mometasone furoate
Natrilix	indapamide
Nerisone	diflucortolone
Nexium	esomeprazole
Nizoral	ketoconazole
Nootropil	piracetam

Nurofen	ibuprofen
Nu-Seals	aspirin
Oilatum	light liquid paraffin, white soft paraffin
Optrex	witch hazel
Orelox	cefpodoxime
Ortho-Gynest	estriol
Oruvail	ketoprofen
Otosporin	hydrocortisone, neomycin, polymyxin
Otrivine	xylometazoline
Panoxyl	benzoyl peroxide
Pariet	rabeprazole
Pevaryl	econazole
Phenergan	promethazine
Picolax	sodium picosulfate, magnesium citrate
Premarin	conjugated oestrogens
Prevenar	pneumococcal polysaccharide conjugate vaccine
Questran	colestyramine
Rasilez	aliskiren
Rennie	calcium carbonate, magnesium carbonate
Rhinocort Aqua	budesonide
Risperdal	risperidone
Roaccutane	isotretinoin
Rocephin	ceftriaxone
Rotarix	live attenuated rotavirus vaccine
Rynacrom	sodium cromoglicate
Senokot	sennosides
Serenace	haloperidol
Slow-K	potassium chloride
Sofradex	dexamethasone, framycetin, gramicidin
Sporanox	itraconazole

Stemetil	prochlorperazine
Stilnoct	zolpidem
Stugeron	cinnarizine
Suboxone	buprenorphine, naloxone
Sudafed	pseudoephedrine
Sudocrem	benzyl alcohol, benzyl benzoate, benzyl cinnamate, lanolin, zinc oxide
Synalar	fluocinolone
Syndol	paracetamol, codeine, caffeine, doxylamine
Tavanic	levofloxacin
Tagamet	cimetidine
Tegretol	carbamazepine
Telfast	fexofenadine
Tenormin	atenolol
Tildiem	diltiazem
Timoptol	timolol
Twinrix	inactivated hepatitis A virus, hepatitis B surface antigen
Uniflu	paracetamol, diphenhydramine, phenylephrine, codeine, caffeine, ascorbic acid
Utinor	norfloxacin
Valium	diazepam
Varilrix	Varicella zoster live-attenuated vaccine
Vasogen	dimeticone, calamine, zinc oxide
Ventolin	salbutamol
Vermox	mebendazole
Viagra	sildenafil
Voltarol	diclofenac
Xalatan	latanoprost
Xenical	orlistat
Xylocaine	lidocaine (lignocaine)
Xyzal	levocetirizine
Yasmin	ethinylestradiol, drospirenone

Zaditen	ketotifen
Zantac	ranitidine
Zestril	lisinopril
Zinnat	cefuroxime
Zithromax	azithromycin
Zocor	simvastatin
Zofran	ondansetron
Zovirax	aciclovir

Appendix B

Definitions of conditions

Acne: skin disease occurring in the presence of sebaceous glands

Acute laryngotracheobronchitis: viral croup

Agranulocytosis: a drastic reduction in the white blood cell count

Allergic rhinitis: hay fever, inflammation of the nasal pathways

Alopecia: hair loss

Amenorrhoea: absence of menstruation

Angina: thoracic pain due to lack of oxygen supply to the myocardium

Anorexia: loss of appetite

Aphthous ulceration: canker sores, mouth sores

Arrhythmias: deviation in the pattern of heartbeat

Arthritis: inflammatory condition of the joints

Ascites: accumulation of fluid in the abdomen

Asthenia: loss of energy

Ataxia: inability to coordinate movements

Attention deficit hyperactivity disorder: affecting children, problems with sustained attention, concentration and task persistence, presenting with overactivity

Blepharitis: inflammation of the hair follicles and the meibomian glands of the eyelids

Bradycardia: heart rate less than 60 beats/min

Bronchodilatation: widening of the bronchi

Bulimia: food craving with overeating followed by purging

Calluses: hard skin occurring in areas prone to pressure or friction

Candidiasis: infection caused by *Candida* species

Cardiotoxicity: toxic effect to the cardiac tissues

Cataract: loss of transparency of the lens of the eye

Chilblains: areas of the skin that are inflamed and present as bluish-red in colour

Chloasma: skin pigmentation of the face occurring during pregnancy or with the use of oral contraceptives

Cholestasis: blocking of the bile pathway in the biliary system

Coeliac disease: inability to metabolise gluten

Cold sores: infection caused by herpes simplex virus

Conjunctivitis: inflammation of the conjunctiva

Contact dermatitis: skin irritation resulting from exposure to a sensitising antigen

Corns: mass of epithelial cells occurring over a bony prominence

Cradle cap: seborrhoeic dermatitis of the scalp occurring in infants

Crohn's disease: inflammatory disease of the gastrointestinal tract

Croup: viral infection of the upper respiratory tract occurring in infants

Cystitis: urinary tract bacterial infection

Dermatitis: inflammation of the skin

Diverticular disease: inflammation of diverticula

Ductus arteriosus: an opening in the fetal heart, which normally closes after birth, joining the pulmonary artery to the aorta

Dyspepsia: epigastric discomfort

Dysphagia: difficulty in swallowing

Dyspnoea: distress in breathing

Dysuria: painful urination

Eczema: skin dermatitis of unknown aetiology

Endometriosis: a condition characterised by growth of endometrial tissue outside the endometrium

Epidural analgesia: anaesthetic injected into the epidural space

Erythema: skin inflammation

Furuncles: boil, staphylococcal infection of a gland or hair follicle

Gastroenteritis: inflammatory condition of the stomach

Gingival hyperplasia: gum tissue overgrowth

Glaucoma: a raised intraocular pressure

Gout: increased uric acid resulting in sodium urate crystals deposited in the joints

Gynaecomastia: enlargement of one or both breasts in male

Haemorrhoids: varicosity in the lower gastrointestinal tract, specifically the rectum or anus

Heart failure: heart does not meet the requirements of the body and the pumping action is less than required

Hiatus hernia: protrusion of a portion of the stomach into the thorax through the oesophageal hiatus of the diaphragm

Hirsutism: excessive body hair in a masculine pattern

Hypercalcaemia: increased calcium blood level

Hyperglycaemia: high blood glucose level

Hyperhidrosis: increased perspiration

Hyperkalaemia: increased plasma potassium level

Hyperkeratosis: growth of keratinised tissue

Hypernatraemia: increased sodium blood level

Hypertension: increased blood pressure

Hyperthyroidism: increased activity of the thyroid gland

Hypoglycaemia: low blood glucose level

Hypokalaemia: low plasma potassium level

Hypothyroidism: decreased activity of the thyroid gland

Impetigo: skin infection

Iritis: inflammation of the iris

Ischaemic heart disease: diminished oxygen supply in the myocardial tissue cells

Ketonuria: excessive amounts of ketone bodies in the urine

Maculopapular eruptions: skin condition characterised by a rash consisting of distinct eruptions

Mania: psychiatric disorder characterised by agitation and elated mood

Multiple sclerosis: progressive degenerative disease presenting with disseminated demyelination of nerve fibres of the brain and spinal cord

Myalgia: muscle pain

Myasthenia gravis: a condition presenting with chronic fatigue and muscle weakness

Myocardial infarction: ischaemia in the cardiac muscle leading to necrosis occurring as a result of reduction in coronary blood flow

Nappy rash: irritation in the napkin area, napkin dermatitis

Nephrotoxicity: toxic to the kidneys

Neural tube defects: congenital malformations of the skull and spinal cord resulting from failure of the neural tube to close during pregnancy

Nocturia: excessive urination at night

Oedema: accumulation of fluid in interstitial spaces

Onychomycosis: fungal nail infections

Osteoarthritis: arthritis associated with degenerative changes of the joints

Osteoporosis: loss of bone density

Otitis externa: inflammation or infection of the external ear

Otitis interna: labyrinthitis, inflammation or infection of the inner ear

Otitis media: inflammation or infection of the middle ear

Paget's disease: non-metabolic disease of the bones

Paraesthesia: numbness and tingling sensation

Parkinson's disease: progressive degenerative neurological disease characterised by tremors and muscle rigidity

Periodontitis: inflammation of the periodontium

Peripheral neuropathies: disorders of the peripheral nervous system

Polycystic ovary syndrome: endocrine disorder characterised by amenorrhoea, hirsutism and infertility

Porphyria: inherited disorders presenting with increased production of porphyrins in the bone marrow

Prostatic hyperplasia: enlargement of the prostate

Pseudomembranous colitis: diarrhoea occurring in patients who received antibacterial agents, caused by the resulting overgrowth of anaerobic bacteria in the gastrointestinal tract

Psoriasis: chronic skin condition presenting with red areas covered with dry, silvery scales

Rhabdomyolysis: injury to muscle tissue

Rhinorrhoea: watery nasal discharge

Rosacea: chronic presentation of acne in adults characterised by dilation of the blood vessels of the face resulting in a flushed appearance

Seborrhoeic dermatitis: chronic inflammatory skin condition

Septicaemia: presence of pathogenic microorganisms or their toxins in the bloodstream

Shingles: herpes zoster, infection due to the re-activation of the latent varicella zoster virus

Status epilepticus: occurrence of continuous seizures

Striae: scars in the skin

Tachycardia: heart rate more than 100 beats/min

Tardive dyskinesia: uncontrollable facial movements

Thrombocytopenia: a reduction in platelet count

Tics: repetitive involuntary movements

Tinea corporis: ringworm infection

Tinea pedis: athlete's foot

Tinnitus: perception of sound such as buzzing, hissing or pulsating noises in the ears

Trigeminal neuralgia: pain and spasms along the trigeminal facial nerve

Typhoid fever: a bacterial infection caused by *Salmonella typhi*

Ulcerative colitis: chronic inflammatory disease affecting the large intestine and the rectum

Urticaria: a skin condition characterised by pruritus

Uterine fibroids: fibrous tissue growth in the uterus

Verrucas: viral skin infection, wart

Appendix C

Abbreviations and acronyms

5HT$_1$ agonist	serotonin receptor agonist type 1
5HT$_3$ antagonist	serotonin receptor antagonist type 3
ACE	angiotensin converting enzyme
ADHD	attention deficit hyperactivity disorder
AV node	atrioventricular node
BCG vaccine	Bacillus Calmette-Guerin vaccine
b.d.	twice daily
CAPD	continuous ambulatory peritoneal dialysis
CBC	complete blood count (full blood count)
CD	controlled drug
COPD	chronic obstructive pulmonary disease
COX-2 inhibitors	cyclo-oxygenase-2 inhibitors
CTZ	chemoreceptor trigger zone
FBC	full blood count
H$_2$-receptor	histamine type 2 receptor
HDL	high density lipoprotein
HER2	human epidermal growth factor receptor-2
HMG CoA	3-hydroxy-3-methylglutaryl coenzyme A
INR	international normalised ratio
LDL	low density lipoprotein
m.	send, prepare
MAOI	monoamine oxidase inhibitor
NIDDM	non-insulin dependent diabetes mellitus
nocte	at night
NSAID	non-steroidal anti-inflammatory drug
o.d.	daily
o.m.	in the morning
o.n.	at night
OTC	over-the-counter preparation
p.c.	after food
PMH	past medical history
PND	paroxysmal nocturnal dyspnoea
p.r.n.	as required

q.d.s.	four times daily
RICE	rest, ice, compression and elevation
RIMA	reversible monoamine oxidase inhibitor type A
rINN	recommended International Non-proprietary Name
SPF	sun protection factor
SSRI	selective serotonin re-uptake inhibitor
TCA	tricyclic antidepressant
t.d.s.	three times daily
UVA	ultraviolet irradiation, long wavelengths
UVB	ultraviolet irradiation, medium wavelengths
w/v	weight in volume
w/w	weight in weight

Appendix D

Performance statistics

The tests were undertaken by a sample of final-year pharmacy students following a five-year course, which included the pre-registration period. The percentage of students answering a question incorrectly is indicated for each test. Questions that were answered correctly by all students are not listed.

Test 1 (n = 36)

Question number	Students answering incorrectly (%)
1	21
2	22
3	28
4	6
6	25
7	25
8	22
10	11
11	28
13	14
14	3
15	53
16	31
17	3
18	14
19	24
21	14
22	3
23	22
25	3
26	3

Test 1 (n = 36) (continued)

Question number	Students answering incorrectly (%)
27	6
28	17
29	6
30	3
31	8
32	6
33	3
34	11
39	6
41	3
44	19
45	6
50	44
51	35
52	15
53	74
54	65
55	8
56	11
57	39
58	61
59	33
60	6
61	64
62	69
64	59
65	19
66	8
67	3
68	6
69	19
70	14

Test 1 (n = 36) (continued)

Question number	Students answering incorrectly (%)
71	8
72	19
73	44
74	22
75	19
76	8
77	8
78	11
79	11
80	17
81	3
82	11
83	25
84	28
85	31
86	72
87	8
88	8
89	3
90	14
91	3
92	39
93	11
94	17
95	11
96	31
97	44
98	3
99	22
100	11

Test 2 (n = 28)

Question number	Students answering incorrectly (%)
2	39
3	39
4	14
5	4
6	54
7	7
8	39
9	18
10	7
11	4
12	21
14	4
15	71
16	75
17	32
18	18
19	7
21	21
23	14
25	32
26	14
27	18
28	7
29	4
30	68
31	4
32	7
33	7
34	32
39	39

Test 2 (n = 28) (continued)

Question number	Students answering incorrectly (%)
40	18
49	82
50	82
51	11
52	82
53	43
54	11
55	4
56	36
57	14
58	11
59	18
60	18
61	18
62	7
63	36
64	14
65	36
66	89
67	38
68	46
69	21
70	39
71	39
72	14
73	7
74	21
75	11
76	32
77	4
78	54
79	25

Test 2 (n = 28) (continued)

Question number	Students answering incorrectly (%)
80	41
81	38
82	68
83	53
84	57
85	61
86	11
87	86
88	36
89	4
90	11
91	59
92	85
93	38
94	88
95	4
96	68
97	39
98	61
99	7
100	32

Test 3 (n = 32)

Question number	Students answering incorrectly (%)
1	6
2	3
4	34
5	3

Test 3 (n = 32) (continued)

Question number	Students answering incorrectly (%)
6	6
7	3
9	65
11	6
12	3
14	13
15	3
17	47
18	13
19	12
20	18
21	38
22	24
23	53
24	9
26	22
27	13
29	9
30	34
31	3
32	53
33	29
34	24
35	3
36	56
37	16
38	28
39	25
40	28
41	6
42	25
43	6
44	13

Test 3 (n = 32) (continued)

Question number	Students answering incorrectly (%)
45	19
46	3
47	13
48	41
49	9
50	28
51	19
52	22
53	31
54	6
55	47
56	6
57	6
58	3
59	41
60	13
61	38
62	19
63	28
65	24
66	44
67	28
68	31
69	3
70	9
79	75
72	9
73	6
74	9
75	56
76	25
77	53
78	9

Test 3 (n = 32) (continued)

Question number	Students answering incorrectly (%)
79	3
80	25
81	62
82	50
83	21
84	41
85	68
86	62
87	56
88	44
89	6
90	13
91	25
92	62
93	50
94	32
95	3
99	19
100	6

Test 4 (n = 26)

Question number	Students answering incorrectly (%)
1	76
2	71
3	35
4	35
5	46
6	8

Test 4 (n = 26) (continued)

Question number	Students answering incorrectly (%)
7	12
8	8
9	8
10	8
11	8
12	4
13	12
15	4
16	19
17	8
18	50
19	31
20	35
21	38
22	31
23	31
24	15
25	23
26	4
27	12
28	27
29	23
30	38
31	12
32	31
33	27
34	23
35	35
36	19
37	62
38	81
39	19

Test 4 (n = 26) (continued)

Question number	Students answering incorrectly (%)
40	42
41	62
42	27
43	23
44	4
45	8
46	27
47	62
48	12
49	77
50	31
51	35
52	69
53	50
54	15
55	46
56	15
57	8
58	62
59	31
60	54
61	42
62	19
63	50
64	69
65	81
66	62
67	62
68	35
69	23
70	46
71	62

Test 4 (n = 26) (continued)

Question number	Students answering incorrectly (%)
72	50
73	58
74	50
75	50
76	54
77	54
78	62
79	38
80	46
81	46
82	69
83	50
84	69
85	4
86	15
87	12
88	15
89	15
90	38
91	31
92	19
93	35
94	38
95	54
96	54
97	15
98	4
99	4

Test 5 (n = 36)

Question number	Students answering incorrectly (%)
1	8
2	17
3	69
4	11
6	17
7	17
8	3
9	61
10	14
11	8
13	24
14	6
15	17
16	6
17	3
18	6
19	33
20	18
21	25
23	31
24	72
25	22
26	3
27	36
28	9
29	14
30	31
31	64
32	14

Test 5 (n = 36) (continued)

Question number	Students answering incorrectly (%)
33	8
34	25
35	14
36	11
37	42
38	42
39	3
40	28
41	6
44	3
45	14
46	3
47	6
48	22
49	3
50	6
51	11
52	33
53	6
54	19
55	58
56	64
57	8
58	8
59	97
60	47
61	3
62	47
63	39
64	47
65	92
66	14

Test 5 (n = 36) (continued)

Question number	Students answering incorrectly (%)
67	19
68	47
69	6
70	3
71	22
73	22
74	6
75	78
76	25
77	83
78	17
80	78
81	11
82	50
83	6
84	61
87	19
88	3
89	11
90	24
91	24
92	12
93	81
94	44
96	8
97	25
98	17
99	56
100	64

Test 6 (n = 28)

Question number	Students answering incorrectly (%)
1	7
2	50
3	29
4	43
5	43
6	43
7	18
8	4
9	50
10	14
11	50
12	11
13	29
14	7
15	14
16	38
18	4
20	11
21	18
22	18
23	43
24	61
25	14
26	7
27	7
28	12
29	4
31	93
32	11
33	18

Test 6 (n = 28) (continued)

Question number	Students answering incorrectly (%)
34	36
35	11
36	14
38	21
42	14
43	21
45	4
46	32
48	4
49	36
50	46
51	14
52	14
53	4
54	82
55	11
56	11
57	21
58	61
59	18
60	18
61	7
62	82
63	32
64	29
65	50
66	46
67	7
68	21
69	25
70	11
71	18

Test 6 (n = 28) (continued)

Question number	Students answering incorrectly (%)
72	50
73	4
74	21
75	79
76	12
77	86
78	43
79	96
80	57
81	68
82	14
83	7
84	89
85	26
86	53
87	29
88	88
89	26
90	38
91	11
92	29
93	25
94	11
95	11
96	56
97	47
98	68
99	74
100	62

Test 7 (n = 32)

Question number	Students answering incorrectly (%)
1	31
2	9
3	25
4	3
5	19
6	6
7	6
8	13
10	13
11	19
12	3
13	59
14	41
17	66
22	9
23	13
25	13
27	3
29	3
30	16
32	16
33	38
34	4
36	3
37	22
38	38
42	78
43	10
44	22
45	22

Test 7 (n = 32) (continued)

Question number	Students answering incorrectly (%)
46	16
47	10
49	31
54	3
55	25
56	3
57	13
61	3
62	59
63	63
64	66
65	10
66	3
67	6
68	28
69	44
71	41
72	13
73	31
74	44
75	9
76	44
77	19
78	31
79	22
80	50
81	3
82	25
83	25
85	3
86	69
87	31

Test 7 (n = 32) (continued)

Question number	Students answering incorrectly (%)
88	22
89	28
90	53
91	66
92	31
93	28
94	3
95	3
96	59
97	9
98	38
99	31
100	13

Test 8 (n = 26)

Question number	Students answering incorrectly (%)
1	12
2	38
4	12
6	4
7	50
8	27
9	27
10	58
11	50
12	8
13	8

Test 8 (n = 26) (continued)

Question number	Students answering incorrectly (%)
14	19
15	69
16	23
17	8
18	12
19	23
21	8
22	12
23	4
24	19
25	12
26	58
27	12
28	31
29	42
30	58
31	46
32	54
33	96
34	73
35	65
36	62
37	77
38	73
39	65
40	23
41	65
42	23
43	23
44	54
45	77
46	31

Test 8 (n = 26) (continued)

Question number	Students answering incorrectly (%)
47	31
48	38
49	27
50	46
51	62
52	23
53	31
54	58
55	31
56	38
57	65
58	35
59	50
60	62
61	73
62	19
63	85
64	31
65	54
66	58
67	62
68	12
69	38
70	23
71	12
72	46
73	15
74	50
75	62
76	58
78	77
79	62

Test 8 (n = 26) (continued)

Question number	Students answering incorrectly (%)
80	4
81	27
83	27
84	35
86	35
87	19
88	4
89	19
90	73
91	65
92	50
93	77
94	58
95	35
96	19
97	92
98	92
99	81
100	54

Proprietary names index

Generic names index

Conditions index

Subject index